CW00733821

# Veterinary Practice Management

# Veterinary Practice Management

**Catherine R. Coates**

*MA(Ed), PG Cert Business Administration, PGCE DipIT(Open), CVPM*
*University of Bristol, UK*

With contributions from

**Alan Jones**

*BSc(Hons), RODP, NEBOSH Cert*

and

**Michael W. Coates**

*BSc(Hons) Forensic Computing*

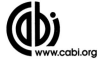
www.cabi.org

CABI is a trading name of CAB International

| | |
|---|---|
| CABI | CABI |
| Nosworthy Way | 38 Chauncey Street |
| Wallingford | Suite 1002 |
| Oxfordshire OX10 8DE | Boston, MA 02111 |
| UK | USA |
| | |
| Tel: +44 (0)1491 832111 | Tel: +1 800 552 3083 (toll free) |
| Fax: +44 (0)1491 833508 | Tel: +1 (0)617 395 4051 |
| E-mail: info@cabi.org | E-mail: cabi-nao@cabi.org |
| Website: www.cabi.org | |

© C.R. Coates 2012. All rights reserved. No part of this publication may be reproduced in any form or by any means, electronically, mechanically, by photocopying, recording or otherwise, without the prior permission of the copyright owners.

A catalogue record for this book is available from the British Library, London, UK.

**Library of Congress Cataloging-in-Publication Data**

Coates, Catherine R.
  Veterinary practice management / by Catherine R. Coates ; with contributions from Alan Jones and Michael W. Coates.
     p. ; cm.
  Includes bibliographical references and index.
  ISBN 978-1-84593-980-9 (alk. paper)
  I. Jones, Alan, BSc. II. Coates, Michael W. III. C.A.B. International. IV. Title.
  [DNLM: 1. Veterinary Medicine–economics. 2. Practice Management. 3. Veterinary Medicine–organization administration. SF 756.4]

636.0890068--dc23

2012021013

ISBN-13: 978 1 84593 980 9

Commissioning editor: Sarah Hulbert
Editorial assistant: Alexandra Lainsbury
Production editor: Simon Hill

Typeset by SPi, Pondicherry, India
Printed and bound by Gutenberg Press, Malta

# Contents

# Preface

The teaching of business management in UK veterinary schools is rapidly becoming established as more schools incorporate business units and modules into their programmes. The relevance of including business management within rather crowded veterinary curricula has been questioned by those who argue that for at least the first five years after graduating, newly qualified veterinarians and veterinary nurses are likely to be entirely focused on improving their clinical knowledge and skills, with little time for management or business. While it is right and proper that clinical aspects should be their primary focus, all too soon they will find themselves conducting discussions with their employers about their work performance and contribution to practice revenues, and how the results that they achieve relate to their pay and other rewards. Newly qualified veterinarians will almost immediately find themselves in charge of staff – nurses, technicians and receptionists – and while teamwork may be the order of the day, they will nevertheless be expected to demonstrate leadership and organizational skills from the start. Equally, veterinary nurses require business knowledge and management skills in order to progress to head nurse or practice manager positions.

Veterinary practice owners and managers require a considerable breadth of business knowledge, which encompasses the disciplines of marketing, human resource management, employment law, finance and systems, among others. The aim of this book is to provide a selection of key topics, which is by no means exhaustive, but which should provide a solid starting point for further study. The treatment of each topic aims to be academic and draws on a range of sources and research which provide an evidence-based rationale for the day-to-day practice of management. Although primarily aimed at undergraduate veterinary and veterinary nursing students, the contents of this book will also be of interest to anyone involved in veterinary practice management in whatever capacity.

The traditional sole-owner and partnership business models, which have predominated until recently, are rapidly being replaced by more complex entities such as joint venture partnerships, franchises and corporates. Veterinary graduates will need to be able to make sense of this complexity and to understand how their particular practice operates as a business if they are to make a meaningful contribution to its success. Providing a sound education in veterinary practice management will enable them to do this.

In the absence of a commonly agreed syllabus for veterinary practice management teaching, each veterinary school will inevitably develop its own content and approach. The University of Bristol has taught veterinary practice management to undergraduate veterinary nursing students for the past 10 years and has gained considerable experience in delivering such teaching. This textbook has grown from the experience so gained.

Catherine R. Coates
*Teaching Fellow in Veterinary Practice Management*

# Introduction
# The Context of Veterinary Practice

The environment within which veterinary practices operate today is complex and ever changing. Managers are continuously facing new challenges, not the least of which is how to ensure survival in the current economic climate.

There are many external influences that have an impact on businesses in a variety of ways. These influences can be grouped into six key external environmental factors – Political, Economic, Sociological, Technological, Legal and Environmental (acronym – PESTLE). Large organizations continuously monitor these factors in an organized way as part of their strategic planning processes. The purpose of this activity is to gauge present and future trends that are likely to be influential and to identify specific challenges and opportunities arising from these. In today's highly competitive environment, this is meant to give organizations an edge over their competitors. But, as recent economic developments have demonstrated, such environmental scanning appears to be more effective as a tool for gauging the *present* climate than it is as a means of predicting the future.

In order to identify and define the external context within which veterinary practices function, it is necessary to make a distinction between the immediate or near environment and the more distant or far environment. The immediate environment comprises a practice's key stakeholders and all other individuals and organizations with which a practice interacts every day. Through these interactions a practice can influence the immediate environment as well as be influenced by it, and so the relationship is a reciprocal one.

The more distant far environment comprises the PESTLE factors identified earlier, both national and global. Individually, veterinary practices may have little or no control over these factors, but collectively, as an industry, they are able to exert some degree of influence (Fig. I.1).

Many of the decisions that business owners and managers make are either determined or are influenced by both the near and far environments. Managers are constantly engaged in balancing the often conflicting needs and interests of stakeholders while at the same time dealing with the threats and opportunities presented by influential factors in the far environment.

The near environment is examined in detail in the forthcoming chapters of this book. Before proceeding, however, let us consider the impact of specific PESTLE factors that are currently exerting an influence on veterinary practices in the UK.

## Political and Legal Factors

Veterinary practices, like all organizations, have to comply with a whole raft of legislation, which comes from both the national government and the European Union (EU), and which determines how organizations conduct their operations. Table I.1 summarizes some of the key legislation that is currently in place, as it applies to the different administrative functions of a business.

This legislation requires implementation, monitoring and control, the cost of which is considerable. Legislation is also constantly changing, so managers must ensure that they keep up to date and that they act promptly when required, as the financial penalties for non-compliance can be prohibitive.

The government also determines levels of taxation and can vary these as it deems necessary, leaving businesses not only with the task of reorganizing their processes to accommodate the changes, but also of justifying to clients any ensuing price increases.

## Economic Factors

The state of the economy affects every aspect of business – the level of demand for veterinary services, the availability of capital for investment, interest rates and the supply of goods and services.

© C.R. Coates 2012. *Veterinary Practice Management* (C.R. Coates)

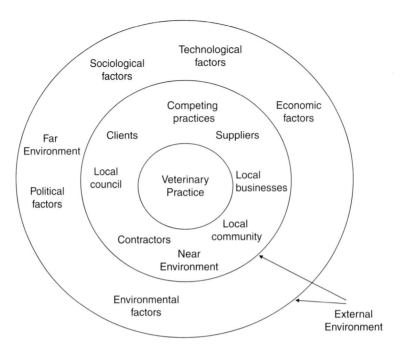

**Fig. I.1.** The external environment.

The current declining economy means that individuals are spending less and consequently businesses are earning less. The increasing cost of fuel, energy and supplies increases costs for businesses. Veterinary practices are having to work hard to control their expenditure, but must also pass on some of these increases to their clients.

The excessive costs of borrowing, combined with low interest rates payable on money invested make it imperative for practices to ensure good cash flows, which are more difficult to achieve when many clients are losing their jobs or suffering pay freezes or cuts and are unable to pay their bills. As a result, more and more practices are introducing payment schemes and savings plans, which allow clients to spread the cost over a longer period of time. These schemes and plans have to be appropriately administered, however, thus leading to an increased administrative burden for practice managers and administrators. Some schemes also require licensing by the Financial Services Authority (FSA).

## Sociological Factors

In the UK, the Pet Food Manufacturers Association (PFMA) commissions annual surveys of the UK pet population. According to the results of the 2011 survey, one in two households owns a pet, which is a high level of pet ownership. However, pet ownership is declining overall, and this is having a noticeable negative impact on practice revenues (VetSupport+, 2010). A comparison of the 2009 and 2011 PFMA survey results (PFMA, 2011) bears this out:

PFMA pet ownership survey results: percentage of households owning a pet (most popular type).

| Type of pet | 2009 | 2011 |
| --- | --- | --- |
| Dog | 23% | 22% |
| Cat | 20% | 18% |
| Indoor fish | 10% | 9% |
| Outdoor fish | 8% | 6% |

PFMA, UK Pet Food Manufacturers Association.

Declining birth and death rates mean that the UK population is ageing. According to a report by The London School of Economics and Political Science (LSE, 2010), the number of people over 65 in the UK will increase by 6.1 million to 15.8 million by the year 2031. This increase is, apparently, progressing at five times the pace of that of the preceding 25 years. The report also predicts that in 2017 older

**Table I.1.** A summary of current UK legislation.

| Computers/Information Technology | Human Resource Management | Marketing/Customer Care | Health and Safety | Finance |
|---|---|---|---|---|
| Copyright, Design and Patents Act 1988 | Employment Rights Act 1996 | Trade Descriptions Act 1968 | The Health and Safety at Work Act 1974 | Consumer Credit Act 1974 |
| The Computer Misuse Act 1990 | National Minimum Wage Act 1998 | Sale of Goods Act 1979 | Health and Safety (First Aid) Regulations 1981 | Value Added Tax Act 1994 (and subsequent Acts) |
| European Council Directive 1991, leading to (UK) Copyright (Computer Programs) Regulations 1992 | Working Time Regulations 1998 | Consumer Protection Act 1987 | Controlled Waste Regulations 1992 | Finance Act 2000 et seq. (updated annually) |
| Health and Safety (Display Screen Equipment Regulations) 1992 | Working Time (Amendment) Regulations 2001 and 2002 | Control of Misleading Advertisements Regulations 1988 | Manual Handling Operations Regulations 1992 | Financial Services and Markets Act 2000 |
| Data Protection Act 1998 | Employment Act 2002 | Sale and Supply of Goods Act 1994 | The Health and Safety at Work Regulations 1992 | The Income Tax (Pay as You Earn) Regulations 2003 (and subsequent annual updates) |
| Regulation of Investigatory Powers Act 2000 (RIPA) | Part-Time Workers Regulations (Prevention of Less Favourable Treatment) 2002 | Sale and Supply of Goods to Consumers Regulations 2002 | Reporting of Injuries, Diseases and Dangerous Occurrences Regulations (RIDDOR) 1995 | Consumer Credit Act 2006 (amends the 1974 Act) |
| Telecoms (Lawful Business Practice) (Interception of Communications) Regulations 2000 | Employment Equality (Age) Regulations 2006 | Control of Misleading Advertisements (Amendment) Regulations 2003 | Special Waste Regulations 1996 | The Companies Act 2006 |
| Freedom of Information Act 2005 | Equality Act 2010 | Consumer Credit (Advertisements) Regulations 2004 | Ionising Radiation Regulations 1999 | |
| | | Veterinary Medicines Regulations 2005 | The Management of Health and Safety at Work Regulations 1999 | |
| | | | The Disability Discrimination (Providers of Services) (Adjustment of Premises) Regulations 2001 | |
| | | | Control of Substances Hazardous to Health (COSHH) Regulations 2002 | |
| | | | Personal Protective Equipment Regulations 2002 | |

people will make up nearly 19% of the total population. Alongside this, due to the economic recession, company pension schemes have either collapsed, have been severely eroded or are undergoing radical reorganization, with employers being forced to reconsider the level of their contributions to these schemes. The government has also extended the state retirement age, with further extensions planned for both men and women to be implemented in stages, which means that a state pension will no longer be available to retirees at age 65. It is likely that a significant proportion of individuals who retire over the next 10–15 years will do so without adequate financial provision in place for their old age, leading inevitably to declining levels of pet ownership and less disposable income to spend on veterinary care.

The demographic profile of the veterinary profession is also changing. In the UK, the number of female veterinarians is increasing dramatically, with females currently significantly outnumbering males in the 25–40 year age group (RCVS, 2011). Veterinary school admission statistics indicate that this trend is likely to continue for the foreseeable future (Fearon, 2011). The gender shift is likely to have a profound effect on the profession. With women still taking primary responsibility for the care of children and elderly dependants in the home, the demand for more family-friendly ways of working, such as part-time working hours, flexible working and other, supportive working patterns (e.g. term-time only, 9 a.m. to 3 p.m.) is likely to increase. This will have implications for the provision of continuity of care and may adversely affect practice standards of client care and communication, and practice revenues. Practices are already having to establish new working patterns that fulfil the needs of staff without compromising the quality of veterinary care being provided.

## Technological Factors

ICT (information and communications technology) eliminates barriers – time and place are now only minor considerations when it comes to accessing information, products, services and other resources. Clients now have a choice of whether to purchase their pets' medicines from their veterinarian or the local pharmacy, or from an online store – which is able to supply prescription drugs more cheaply than the veterinarian. Thus competition in pricing and supply is increased for practices, a trend which is likely to continue. Practices are, therefore, strengthening their Internet presence and setting up e-commerce facilities as well as using social networking sites as a means of retaining their existing clients.

Practice management systems are likely to continue to develop and evolve as vendors strive to pre-empt practice needs and produce new solutions for problems that practices do not even know they yet have. So the pressure to upgrade systems is enormous, despite the considerable cost.

Continuing advances in human and veterinary medicine mean that diagnostic and surgical equipment and instruments are becoming more and more sophisticated, and more affordable, requiring that veterinarians and nurses continue to remain at the cutting edge in terms of both skills and knowledge. Future business strategies will need to include structured plans for replacing equipment and upgrading technology, with budgets set aside to enable these plans to be implemented relatively quickly and easily. Practices will also need to ensure that they manage staff training more proactively, setting aside annual training budgets, which can also be used as a bargaining tool for attracting the best applicants for positions that become vacant.

## Environmental Factors

Pollution control and waste disposal are the main thrust of current environmental legislation, and it is likely that in the not too distant future practices will be required to carry out regular environmental audits and to report on their performance and the steps that they are taking to minimize their impact on the environment. Local communities, clients, employees and local government are likely to take a greater interest in this aspect of a veterinary practice's activities, especially if a practice plans to invest in new premises, or to extend existing or offer new services that require more space and new equipment. With local councils seeking to reduce the number of waste collections from premises, practices will also be forced to consider alternative methods of waste disposal, irrespective of the cost.

Clearly, the macro-environment within which veterinary practices operate exerts a profound and complex influence, which often leads to change. How can practices arm themselves against the negative effects of these influences? One way is to ensure that internal systems and processes are as efficient and effective as possible and that they truly serve the needs of both clients and staff without undue waste and expense. Other ways include:

- being well informed through reading the veterinary press and keeping up to date with local, national and international news
- maintaining membership of professional bodies and associations
- regular attendance at conferences and congresses
- networking with colleagues to share information and ideas
- undertaking continuous training and development.

Change is inevitable and the pace of change is increasing. Veterinary practices will survive only by remaining flexible and adopting a culture of continuous growth and development.

## References

Fearon, R. (2011) Putting gender on the agenda. *Veterinary Times* 41(32), 10–12.

LSE (2010) *Improving Service Delivery to Older People in the UK: Strategies for Local Authorities. A Report Commissioned by Deloitte from The London School of Economics and Political Science.* Available at: http://www.deloitte.com/assets/Dcom-UnitedKingdom/Local%20 Assets/Documents/Industries/GPS/UK_GPS_LSE_ ageing_population.pdf (accessed 30 May 2012).

PFMA (2011) *Pet Ownership Trends 2011.* Pet Food Manufacturers' Association, London. Available at: http://www.pfma.org.uk/pet-ownership-trends/ (accessed 13 March 2012).

RCVS (2011) *RCVS Facts 2011, The Annual Report of The Royal College of Veterinary Surgeons: Part 2.* Royal College of Veterinary Surgeons, London. Available at: http://www.rcvs.org.uk/publications/ rcvs-facts-2011/rcvsfacts2011.pdf (accessed 30 May 2012).

VetSupport+ (2010) *Business Insights: The Changing Veterinary Environment.* Available at: http:// vetsupportplus-co-uk.server5.controldns.co.uk/ environment-article.php (accessed 30 May 2012).

# SECTION 1
# The Practice–Client Relationship (1): Marketing Veterinary Services

**Section Objectives**

At the end of this section, you should be able to:

- Explain the differences between products and services.
- Understand and explain the principles of services marketing.
- Understand how clients perceive service quality.
- Understand the term 'relationship marketing' and explain its relevance to veterinary practice.
- Describe the practice communication mix and how it can be used to improve the practice–client relationship.
- Discuss and apply techniques for building client loyalty.
- Evaluate the costs and benefits of marketing activities.

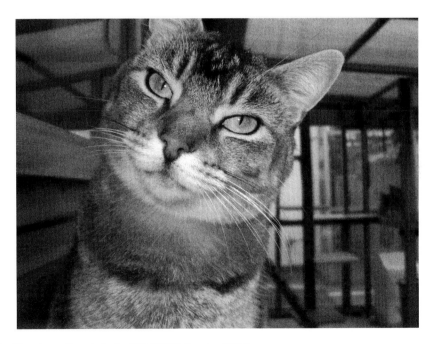

There are 8 million domestic cats in the UK (PFMA Survey, 2011)

# 1 The Characteristics of Services

All businesses, including veterinary practices, must engage in some form of marketing, the basic purpose of which is to draw the attention of the customer to the service or product that is on offer and to keep them coming back for more. Businesses that sell products – tangible items that can be packaged and placed on a shop shelf for sale – will approach this marketing task differently from companies that offer services. This is because services differ from products in a number of important ways, so some marketing tools that work for products may not work for services and vice versa.

Veterinary staff are engaged in providing a service to animals and their owners and are themselves an important marketing tool for the practices in which they work. If they are to provide a quality service, it is vital that they understand from the outset that they are not simply providing their veterinary clinical knowledge and skills, but a 'service package' comprising a range of important additional components, which clients may value almost as much.

Services have four key characteristics that distinguish them from products – intangibility, inseparability, variability and perishability (Jobber, 2001).

## Intangibility

With most products, customers can usually see what they are getting for their money. Products can be seen, touched, tasted or smelled before purchase. Services tend to be sets of actions performed by the service provider, or sets of procedures or information, knowledge or expertise applied to the resolution of a presenting case or a set of circumstances. Knowledge, or expertise, which lies at the centre of services, is a relatively intangible thing. It is often difficult to price a unit of service and thus to explain exactly what its components are. Veterinary services are often complex – if one were to try to price an operation to surgically remove an

intestinal foreign body from a Labrador, for example, by listing all the different tasks undertaken by staff and the consumables used in carrying out this operation, one would end up with a very long list, which may or may not be complete. Despite this intangibility and complexity, clients expect clarity and it is vital that practices seek ways to provide this. One obvious example of an attempt to provide clarity is an itemized bill giving detailed breakdowns of charges, so that clients can see exactly what they are paying for. Of course, products will have intangible elements and services will have tangible elements as part of the package – but it is the predominance of intangible elements that distinguishes a service from a product.

In product marketing, the focus is naturally on the tangibles. So the type and appearance of the packaging are important, as is the overall size, shape, colour and look of the product itself. Suppliers will highlight the features of the product and the benefits that these features bring to the customer. Advertising campaigns will show the product being used or consumed or satisfying an obvious need or matching a particular lifestyle.

The intangible characteristic of services means that clients will tend to look to the tangible cues that are available for an indication of the quality of the service provided. Therefore, they will make judgements about the physical appearance of the practice building, the look, feel, cleanliness and smell of the waiting room, the appearance and professionalism of the staff, and the way the veterinarian treats them and their pets during a consultation. These tangible cues are very important to clients and need to be carefully managed so that they build the desired impression of a quality service. Hoffman and Bateson (1997) recommend that service providers strive to 'tangibilize the intangible'; some of the many ways that this is done in a veterinary practice are listed in Table 1.1.

**Table 1.1.** Providing tangible cues of service quality.

| Cue | Quality message conveyed |
| --- | --- |
| A group photograph of practice staff with their pets on display in the waiting room | The staff in this practice are pet owners themselves, so will understand clients' needs |
| Staff photographs with job titles and qualifications on display in the waiting room | The staff are qualified to treat clients' pets |
| A checklist completed by the vet when carrying out a health check and given to the client afterwards | The pet's health check was thorough and reassuring for the client |
| A detailed breakdown of all procedures carried out and consumables used in an operation with prices – to accompany the bill | The practice is honest and transparent in its dealings with its clients |
| Well-written, informative leaflets on different aspects of pet health available in the waiting room | The practice is the best place to find information on pet health issues |

## Inseparability

With products, there usually is a time lag between manufacture and final consumption because products can be manufactured, stored and then distributed to retailers for sale to customers. Services, in contrast, are produced and consumed simultaneously. For example, the veterinarian will perform a health check on a client's dog while the client looks on, or will perform an operation or a dental procedure on a dog who must receive these as they are being provided. Once services have been performed, they can rarely be undone or returned by the client, although it may be possible for them to be redone by the service provider or corrected in some way subsequently.

Because services are produced and consumed simultaneously, the staff with whom clients come into contact are key to the client's experience of the service. This interaction between the client and staff member is the 'service encounter', during which the way staff behave towards clients, their tone, attitude, conduct and what they say and do will represent the service itself and will have a considerable influence on the degree of satisfaction that a client feels (Blackman, 2006). Because most staff in a veterinary practice have regular contact with clients, it follows that they should possess excellent communication skills and the ability and authority to put clients' needs first when necessary and appropriate. Staff training and development should, therefore, be a priority for management, because well-trained, competent and empowered employees will contribute directly and positively to client satisfaction. Empowerment comes from employees being able to make decisions without having to refer to a higher authority. Employee remuneration should, in turn, reflect the contribution that is being made by individuals to the success of the business.

## Variability

Customers can expect products made by the same manufacturer to be generally of the same quality whichever retailer they buy them from, but they cannot be sure that service quality will be the same every time. Veterinarians who provide the same service can possess differing levels of skill or expertise, or they might differ in their ability to communicate with clients. The careful selection of appropriately qualified staff will minimize the variability of service provision, as will professional standards and a sound programme of staff training and development and staff appraisal. In the UK, the Royal College of Veterinary Surgeons' Practice Standards Scheme, which accredits practices based on a set of carefully devised standards, serves to reassure the public about the quality of the veterinary care that is being provided by practices.

However, it is not always that simple. One client's perceived excellent quality might be another's perceived mediocre quality. Everyone is different and so people's perceptions of the same experience will also differ. Clients have differing expectations. If the gap between expectations and perceived service quality is too great, clients are likely to defect to another practice where the perceived gap is smaller or non-existent. Even though it is difficult to objectively measure these varying perceptions and expectations, practices must attempt to do so, and a way of doing this is to get to know their clients – their needs, preferences, wants and desires. For this, good communication is key, as is creating an atmosphere that fosters openness, the giving and receiving of constructive feedback, and plenty of opportunities for clients to express their views. Clients' views can be sought in a number of different ways – through talking to them directly every day, by conducting client surveys, by holding focus group meetings, and by placing suggestion boxes in the waiting room or complaint monitoring. Good-quality client feedback is invaluable in discovering any gaps in service quality.

Harvey (1998) identifies two broad components of service quality – quality of *results* and quality of the *process* that customers have to go through to obtain the results they want. If a practice is able to make sick pets better consistently and reliably, without any mistakes, then it is providing quality of results. Process quality has two components – objective or technical process quality and perceptual quality. Technical process quality is achieved when all processes and procedures that the customer must go through follow the state of the art in the field. According to Harvey (1998), the perceptual component comprises four generic dimensions:

1. Empathy – the customer perceives that he/she is understood, that staff care and that they are doing the best for his/her pet.
2. Responsiveness – the customer perceives that the service provider gives prompt and efficient service tailored to his/her individual needs.
3. Assurance – the customer perceives that he/she is in safe, able and competent hands.
4. Tangibles – the customer perceives that all the tangible aspects of the service are of a high quality.

Although Harvey's (1998) article is not about veterinary services, these generic dimensions of service provision are useful in that they direct our focus towards what customers essentially want, which is a question that veterinary practices should always be asking.

For veterinary practices, three additional process quality dimensions can be added (Moreau and Nap, 2010):

5. Flexibility – clients perceive that they are able to access veterinary services and products at a time and place convenient to them.
6. Transparency – clients perceive that the practice is open and honest about its charges and costs.
7. Communication – clients perceive that all the information provided to them by the practice is clear and comprehensible.

Practices should aim to satisfy their clients in all of these process quality dimensions. It is argued that a combination of excellent result and process quality leads to satisfied clients and produces a service that is very hard for other practices to compete with.

## Perishability

Products can be stored for varying lengths of time and do not have to be sold straight away, so they have a certain 'shelf life'. Thus stock levels can be changed to match fluctuations in demand – what isn't sold today can be kept and sold another time. Services cannot be stockpiled in the same way and cannot adapt so easily to fluctuations in demand. So an appointment not kept by a client represents money lost, because if it cannot be filled that day, it cannot be kept for another day. Similarly, if a puppy party has to be cancelled at the last minute owing to a lack of demand, this represents staff time and other practice resources wasted.

One way to avoid this wastage is to ask clients to notify of any cancelled appointments at least 48 h in advance. This requirement can be spelled out to all new clients upon registering with the practice as part of the practice–client 'contract'. Other methods include texting clients to remind them of their appointments the day before, having flexible appointment systems that allow clients to book a day and time most convenient to them and extending opening times to evenings, early mornings and Saturdays in order to maximize client choice. Additional tools, such as online appointment booking systems, online repeat prescription requests and product ordering, help to provide the level of choice, convenience and flexibility that clients expect today.

Taking into account these service characteristics, any approach to marketing veterinary services should be based on the following principles:

1. Practices must manage service tangibles carefully in order to convey the correct message about the quality of the veterinary care provided.
2. Client contact staff are crucial to the clients' experience of the service because they represent the service to the client. It is essential to employ well-qualified and experienced personnel with excellent communication skills and to provide a good working environment, empowerment and appropriate remuneration.

**3.** Practices should strive to achieve *both* result and process quality.

**4.** Clients' views of the service provided are essential for improved service delivery. Practices must make efforts to get to know their clients, their wants, needs and desires, and to provide two-way channels of communication, that are always open.

**5.** Practices should strive to accommodate clients' needs for flexibility as far as is practically possible or be prepared to provide compensatory benefits to minimize the negative effects of a lack of flexibility.

## References

Blackman, K. (2006) Managing service delivery. In: *B713 Fundamentals of Senior Management, Block 3, Sessions 11–13.* The Open University, Milton Keynes, UK.

Hoffman, K.D. and Bateson, J.E.G. (1997) *Essentials of Services Marketing.* The Dryden Press Series in Marketing, Dryden Press, Hinsdale, Chicago, Illinois.

Jobber, D. (2001) *Principles and Practice of Marketing,* 3rd edn. McGraw-Hill, Maidenhead, UK.

Harvey, J. (1998) Service quality: a tutorial. *Journal of Operations Management* 16, 583–597.

Moreau, P. and Nap, R.C. (2010) *Essentials of Veterinary Practice: An Introduction to the Science of Practice Management.* Henston Veterinary Publications, Veterinary Business Development, Peterborough, UK.

## Revision Questions

**1.** Select a practice with which you are familiar and identify the ways in which this practice satisfies the seven process quality dimensions described. If you discover some quality gaps, suggest ways in which these might be filled.

**2.** To what extent does your chosen practice follow the five principles of marketing veterinary services given at the end of this chapter?

**3.** Based on your answer to Question 2, decide whether this practice provides excellent service quality.

**4.** List at least ten ways in which your selected practice endeavours to '*tangibilize the intangible*' so that clients understand the quality of the service provided.

# 2 Building the Practice–Client Relationship

The practice–client relationship could potentially last throughout a pet's entire life, but the practice must work hard to build that relationship so that the client wants to and chooses to stay.

Higgins (2010) argues that the best way for practices to remain profitable and to grow is through building a loyal client base. The particular approach to marketing services that is aimed specifically at retaining existing clients rather than gaining new ones is referred to as 'relationship marketing' (Jobber, 2001). A related concept is 'customer bonding' or 'customer loyalty', in which a service provider aims not only to retain existing clients, but also to bind them to the business for the longer term, such that they are completely loyal and always ready to recommend the service provider to others.

Individuals have to experience a service before they can decide whether it is good or not. Selecting a service provider without any prior knowledge of the quality of the service is risky. Prospective clients try to reduce that risk by seeking the opinions of people who have already experienced the service. Loyal clients are more likely to recommend the practice to others and are, therefore, an important marketing tool. Research has shown that there are considerable benefits both for the practice and for its clients in developing a long-term relationship. The practice benefits financially – from continued sales over the lifetime of the pet and from reduced costs, as the marketing effort and expense involved in retaining existing clients is far smaller than that involved in gaining new ones. A mutually beneficial relationship also increases employee satisfaction and retention. For clients, the result is peace of mind, reduction in risk and stress levels, a sense of security and a better quality service that can be personalized to fit their needs (Jobber, 2001).

Higgins (2010) asserts that practices should treat the practice–client interaction as a 'personal relationship' which is founded on trust, compassion and patience. To build a good relationship requires effort on both sides, so while practices must appreciate that their clients have needs, wants and expectations, they can also reasonably expect clients to fulfil their obligations in relation to them. It helps a relationship if the parties involved have something in common, and one can reasonably assume that both the practice and the client want what is best for the animal under their care.

Relationships take time to develop. The process of relationship building has five key elements:

1. Learning about each other
2. Meeting each other's needs
3. Identifying each other's changing perspectives and preferences and being ready to adapt
4. When things go wrong, putting them right as quickly as possible
5. If things cannot be put right, ending the relationship graciously.

## Learning About Each Other: What Clients Want

The practice needs to know what clients want and clients need to know what the practice can do for them. Obviously, clients want a good standard of veterinary care for their pets. In addition to this, they want (Shilcock and Stutchfield, 2008):

- To feel welcome when they come into the practice
- To feel important
- For staff to be friendly, caring and helpful
- To receive individual attention
- To be listened to and treated with respect
- For staff to give them time.

According to Corsan and Mackay (2001), reiterated by Jevring-Bäck and Bäck (2007), clients respond very favourably to practice staff who also:

- Look and behave like professionals
- Are polite and courteous
- Show interest in and enthusiasm for them, their pets and their children
- Show affection to the pet

- Handle the pet kindly and do not use unnecessary restraint
- Give an accurate estimate of fees
- Accept phone calls from clients requesting information and advice.

Moreau and Nap (2010) make a distinction between implicit and explicit client expectations. Explicit expectations are those that clients make clear or spell out, for example: *'Please can you come and have a look at my horse, she is lame again'*, or *'My cat seems to have gone off his usual food, can you suggest an alternative?'*. Implicit expectations are not spelt out, but can be deemed nevertheless to exist, such as an expectation that clients will always be able to get an appointment on a day and at a time convenient to themselves. According to Moreau and Nap (2010), clients' implicit expectations include:

- Availability – no waiting, flexible hours, easy access and parking, sufficient stock
- Transparency – prices should be clearly labelled, invoices should be itemized
- Choice – various products and services, freedom of choice
- Environment – comfortable, neat, clean, odourless, friendly and modern
- Clarity of the offer – prices listed, clear estimates
- Personalization – services adapted to pet owners' specific needs.

Every practice's client base will have different characteristics, so rather than rely on what others say clients want, it is advisable for practices to carry out their own research to find out what their own clients' needs are.

Finding out how clients learnt about the practice in the first place will give some idea of what it is that brings new clients in. One way of doing this is to ask every new client who registers with the practice how they found out about it and what made them choose this practice instead of the one down the road. Moreau and Nap (2010) report the results of a survey carried out in the USA by the American Veterinary Medical Association, which revealed that convenient location was the top deciding factor, followed by word-of-mouth recommendation, then pricing, then hours and availability. However, while convenience may be the deciding factor for clients looking for a practice, it will be the quality of the service provided that will keep them coming back.

Methods that practices commonly use to find out what clients want include:

- Talking to clients
- Questionnaires – online or paper based and either handed to clients to complete while they are waiting to be seen or sent out by email or in the post (now less common)
- Suggestion boxes kept in reception
- Use of external consultants
- Owner panels or practice–client focus groups.

The first three of these are the easiest and cheapest methods, but the response rate to questionnaires tends to be poor, even when an incentive to complete is provided. Questionnaires handed out by the receptionist have a better response rate, so long as the receptionist chooses the moment carefully. Short and simple questionnaires are quick and easy to complete and clients can usually do so while at the same time listening for their names to be called by the veterinarian, but the amount of valuable information that can be obtained in this way is limited. Suggestion boxes tend to be ignored by clients. External consultants, who specialize in marketing and customer care, can use non-intrusive methods (e.g. mystery shoppers), which can produce very useful information, but their true value really lies in the fact that they are seeing the practice for the first time and are able to provide a fresh outsider's view, picking up on things that staff have become desensitized to over time. Of course, there is also a cost involved in using consultants. Practice–client focus groups can work well with an interested and enthusiastic group of clients and staff. The careful selection of group members is crucial – does one select from the pool of loyal, bonded clients or from those clients who only use the practice occasionally, or from a random selection of clients? Should group composition be changed periodically? What incentives should be provided to those clients who participate and give their valuable views? How often should the group meet? What will be the group's remit? All these questions need to be addressed before such a group is set up, so that its purpose is clear.

### Learning About Each Other: What the Practice Can Offer

The other side of the coin is to make sure that clients know what the practice can offer in terms of services, products, support, information, facilities and staff expertise. The process of client 'education' begins on the very first visit when the receptionist runs through the practice's 'terms of business' with the client, detailing payment terms, the amount of notice required for repeat prescriptions or special dietary foods, information on the availability of appointments, opening times, pet insurance and out-of-hours emergency procedures. All of this information would also be available to the client as part of the practice brochure, which is updated periodically following any changes.

Subsequently, the practice has at its disposal a range of communication tools, which it utilizes to keep clients informed. The practice's communication mix is discussed in Chapter 3.

### Meeting Each Other's Needs

Once client needs have been identified, made explicit and are understood by all staff, practices should strive to meet them as far as is practically possible in a way that still allows the practice to make a reasonable profit. However, if a practice is able to exceed a client's expectations and delight them on the first occasion, it is likely that this client will have higher expectations of the next encounter and so, for the same quality of service, they may be merely satisfied rather than delighted second time around (Harvey, 1998). Consequently, practices must maintain a continuous, sustained effort. For this, they need highly motivated staff trained in client communication who are fully aware that their actions directly affect the level of client satisfaction. In order to do their jobs well, staff need to know what is expected of them and should be supported by efficient processes and procedures, and sound policies. The importance of the receptionist cannot be overstated, as the receptionist is the first point of contact for all existing and prospective clients. The selection and retention of good receptionists is crucial to client satisfaction.

Clients should be made aware that they also have a duty to the practice – to arrive for appointments on time, to pay promptly, to explain fully what is wrong with their pet and not to withhold relevant information, to be polite and courteous, to seek clarification, to listen to the instructions for treatment and to comply with them.

### Be Alert to Each Other's Changing Expectations

Establishing a relationship founded on honesty, trust and mutual respect is more likely to result in clients choosing to remain with the practice in the longer term. However, there are no guarantees, because clients will always wish to exercise choice and, inevitably, circumstances and expectations will change over time. Practices should be alert to changes in clients' circumstances and be flexible enough to adapt their services to changing client needs. If a continuous dialogue with clients is maintained, alongside continuous environmental monitoring, practices should remain flexible enough to adapt.

### When Things Go Wrong – Put Them Right as Quickly as Possible

The practice's procedure for handling complaints and mistakes should be open, honest and credible. Every mistake or complaint is an opportunity to learn and to improve the service for the future benefit of clients so that the same mistake is never made twice. Clients should be encouraged to provide feedback on the service being provided. This can be done simply by the receptionist asking '*Is everything alright? Is there anything else I can help you with today?*', or by using more formal methods.

Clients are often reluctant to complain directly to the veterinarian, but as soon as they leave the consulting room, they are able to express their complaint freely to the receptionist. Reasons for complaints are many and varied. Most can be dealt with immediately. More serious complaints, however, should be referred to the appropriate person – the practice manager, practice principal or one of the partners, to investigate. It is advisable that no one involved with the case should investigate it, as the investigation must be seen to be as objective as possible in order to avoid accusations of 'closing ranks' or 'covering up'. The client must be kept informed at all times of the progress of the investigation. If the practice is found to be at fault, it must apologize and offer suitable compensation. Usually a full refund will suffice, but if an animal has died, this may not be sufficient compensation for the loss of a beloved pet.

### Ending the Relationship Graciously

From time to time, the practice–client relationship may well break down completely, despite the practice's best efforts to prevent this. Relationship breakdown can happen for a variety of reasons. Once in a while, clients may feel that their complaint was not dealt with to their satisfaction and may wish to take the matter further. In such instances, the practice should assist the client by providing the contact details of the relevant representative body and by cooperating with any investigation that may subsequently arise.

A common reason for a breakdown in the practice–client relationship is a client's refusal to pay their outstanding veterinary fees. Practices have procedures in place for chasing client debts, but when these prove ineffective, it is reasonable for a practice to refuse further treatment – except in the event of an emergency – but it must first notify the client in writing of its intention to do so.

When a client makes a decision to transfer to another practice, the original practice should ensure that the animal's records are transferred promptly to the new practice upon request. It may be possible to ask the client why they are transferring, which would provide valuable information, but most of the time clients who intend to leave do not give any prior warning and there is not much that a practice can do about this. The loss of one or two clients a year in this way may not be a cause for concern, but if this number begins to rise noticeably, then the practice has a serious problem, which must be investigated and dealt with urgently.

To summarize:

- Successful practice–client relationships are built up over time and are based on trust and mutual respect.
- Both parties must be willing to spend time and effort learning about each other.
- Practices need clients more than clients need them.
- The client will always retain the right to choose and can decide to change at any time.
- The effort put into retaining existing clients must be sustained and continuous.

Even though client loyalty cannot be guaranteed, the ability to satisfy clients' needs consistently and successfully will have a positive impact on practice revenues and client retention rates.

## References

Corsan, J. and Mackay, A.R. (2001) *The Veterinary Receptionist: Essential Skills for Client Care*, 1st edn. Butterworth-Heinemann, Oxford, UK.

Harvey, J. (1998) Service quality: a tutorial. *Journal of Operations Management* 16, 583–597.

Higgins, N. (2010) Back to basics. *Veterinary Management for Today*, March 2010, 14–15. Veterinary Practice Management Association (VPMA), Kettering, UK.

Jevring-Bäck, C. and Bäck, E. (2007) *Managing a Veterinary Practice*, 2nd edn. Saunders Elsevier, Philadelphia, Pennsylvania.

Jobber, D. (2001) *Principles and Practice of Marketing*, 3rd edn. McGraw-Hill, Maidenhead, UK.

Moreau, P. and Nap, R.C. (2010) *Essentials of Veterinary Practice: An Introduction to the Science of Practice Management.* Henston Veterinary Publications, Veterinary Business Development, Peterborough, UK.

Shilcock, M. and Stutchfield, G. (2008) *Veterinary Practice Management: A Practical Guide*, 2nd edn. Saunders Elsevier, Edinburgh, UK.

## Revision Questions

**1.** Drawing on the material in this chapter and at least two other published sources, explain the concept of '*client loyalty*'.

**2.** Explain the reciprocal nature of the practice–client relationship and the responsibilities that each party has towards the other.

**3.** Identify at least three ways in which practices can adapt to changing client expectations.

**4.** A small animal veterinary practice provides services to owners of a number of different species. Discuss the differing needs of dog and cat owners and the provisions that practices make to accommodate these differing needs.

# 3 The Practice Communication Mix

Communication is the means by which practices get to know their clients and build trust. Sharma and Patterson (1999) argue that effective communication is instrumental in generating client trust and developing long-term client relationships. Jevring-Bäck and Bäck (2007) support this view and list communication as one of 'The 7 Cs of Trust', alongside competence, consistency, compassion, costs, cheerfulness and commitment.

There are many and varied ways of communicating with clients, and most practices employ a range of tools and channels. The range of communication activities that a business engages in is called the 'communication mix'. In order to communicate effectively, practices must ensure that the communication mix is integrated and consistent with their overall mission and aims. It is also important to clarify the purpose of all client communications before selecting the medium or method of transmission that is the most appropriate for the message being conveyed.

Research has shown that personalized forms of communication tailored to individual needs are more effective in building good practice–client relationships. Communications that are perceived by clients as personally relevant, useful and worthwhile add value to the service provided, clearly complementing it by giving clients something they actually want so that they are not immediately tempted to throw material in the waste bin as soon as they return home after seeing the veterinarian or as soon as the information arrives in the mailbox. The key to success lies in achieving the right balance of face-to-face or verbal, paper-based and electronic communications.

Figure 3.1 shows a typical communication mix of a small animal practice. While practices will not utilize all of the communication methods shown, most will adopt a scattergun approach without following any specific strategy.

## Communication as Marketing

Clearly, all of these methods of communication are forms of marketing and most of them make up the practice's 'promotional mix'. The 'promotional mix' comprises the following components (Jobber, 2001):

- Advertising – e.g. Yellow Pages, advertisement in local press
- Personal selling – face-to-face communication, e.g. veterinarian or nurse recommending a specific pet diet or flea treatment
- Direct marketing – e.g. annual health check reminders, worming or vaccination reminders
- Internet and online marketing – e.g. repeat prescription requests via practice web site, e-commerce
- Sales promotion – e.g. two-for-one offers, discounts, special promotions
- Publicity – e.g. articles in the local press or on the radio.

Whether a practice chooses to use any one or all of these components will depend on a number of factors:

1. The costs involved – some promotional tools, such as radio or press advertising, can be expensive.
2. The information needs of the clients – there is hardly any point in producing information that clients have no interest in, so most communications should be produced in order to satisfy a clearly identified client need.
3. The skills, experience and enthusiasm of staff – practices rely on their staff – veterinarians, veterinary nurses and receptionists – to 'sell' their services and products, to produce material for newsletters, organize and participate in open days and client talks – in addition to carrying out their professional work. The personal skills of these people, their experience and enthusiasm for such activities will determine how successful they are, as

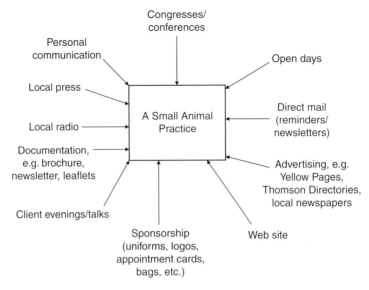

**Fig. 3.1.** A small animal practice communication mix.

well as the level of importance that the practice itself (i.e. its owners) places on such activities.

4. The activities of competitors – very often a practice will be pushed into additional promotional activity in order to keep up with a competitor who has launched a marketing campaign of its own, or a new service or innovative promotion. The fear of losing clients to a competitor is ever present, so practices must be seen to be competitive in their offerings.

Each component of the promotional mix has its advantages and disadvantages, and it is important for those engaged in practice promotion to understand what these are.

## Advertising

Advertising is any form of non-personal communication to clients and potential clients about the practice and its services using a variety of media, such as the Internet, local free publications, newspapers, local cinemas or radio. One clear advantage of advertising is that it can reach a wide audience quickly. Because of this, it can be a cost-effective method of promotion. But its effectiveness in terms of gaining new clients or securing repeat business is difficult to ascertain unless the practice makes an effort to trace the effects of advertising, either by asking new clients how they learnt about the practice or by using promotional codes or

vouchers which clients can bring with them when they next come into the practice. It is not possible to do this with all advertising, however, and nowadays clients are more likely to search the Internet for a local practice or ask their neighbours and friends.

There is no consensus among researchers about how advertising works, because of the variety of uses that it is put to. Page (2009) argues that advertising does work, but that it is persuasive rather than coercive – in other words, it cannot make people buy if they don't want to. Jobber (2001) discusses two predominant groups of theories – *strong and weak theories* of how advertising works. The strong theory is based around the AIDA principle, which claims that potential customers pass through a series of stages – from initial Awareness through an Interest in the product or service, which then turns into a Desire to purchase or a conviction that the product or service is for them and, finally, to Action resulting in a purchase. Proponents of this theory claim that advertising can be as powerful as that and is capable of changing people's attitudes – converting them from non-buyers into buyers. Certainly, examples of such powerful advertising can easily be found – one need only think of the big cosmetics brands, such as L'Oréal or Rimmel, or soft drinks brands, such as Coca Cola and Pepsi, where the purpose of advertising seems to be to establish an entire way of life that incorporates the relevant product or brand. This theory will not apply to all products, though and, specifically with high volume, inexpensive consumer goods, most people are unlikely to feel any strong desire to purchase or any strong conviction that one brand is better than another. This leads to the alternative weak theory of advertising – the ATR model, involving the three steps of Awareness, Trial and Reinforcement – according to which advertising is only capable of arousing curiosity and a possible first trial purchase, which may lead to subsequent purchases if the product is liked. The purpose of advertising in this case is to provide reinforcement and reassurance to buyers that they are making the correct purchasing decision.

Of course, these theories are more applicable to products than to services, but one could argue that the strong theory is more applicable to veterinary services, both because there is a high level of client involvement in the service provided and because interest in the practice and a desire to remain a client need to be very actively built. It is doubtful whether advertising could achieve this on its own, especially as a client's choice of veterinary practice is more often than not guided purely by basic concerns, such as whether the practice is conveniently located or whether there is adequate parking, and how its prices compare with those of competitors.

Two key items of practice literature represent forms of advertising – the practice brochure and the practice newsletter. Practice brochures have been around for a long time and are a good way of providing new and prospective clients with basic information about the practice. Brochures usually contain the following information:

- Opening times
- Contact details
- Details of the facilities and services provided – with pictures
- What to do in the event of an emergency
- Information about key members of staff – practice principal(s) and partners
- Price list.

The drawback of brochures is that they can be expensive to produce and, once they are printed, cannot be changed and may become out of date very quickly. That is why it is best to limit the information provided to those facts which are not likely to change too quickly, or to produce a folder-type brochure with slots inside for separate sheets

containing the information that is subject to change, so that these can easily be updated and replaced. The practice web site is rapidly replacing the practice brochure.

## Practice newsletter

Richardson and Richardson (2010) argue that the practice newsletter is probably the '*most effective client boosting method*' that a practice has at its disposal. They urge practices to spend a lot more time and care in producing their newsletters than they currently do, primarily because the newsletter is a practice's opportunity to actively and regularly present clients with reasons to visit the surgery more often. However practices may view the purpose of newsletters, they must be a good read and they must contain information that clients want, otherwise clients will simply ignore them.

Newsletters will include any or all of the following:

- Latest news and features about the practice
- At least one story about an unusual or successful case
- A diary of forthcoming events and who to contact about them
- One or two staff profiles (existing or new staff)
- Brief details of surgery hours, contact numbers, e-mail address and web site URL
- Information about any improvements planned, changes to premises and new services and products
- Short articles on preventive health care issues with a seasonal slant.

Although it is possible to produce a newsletter in house relatively cheaply, it is essential to get professional advice about layout, design and printing at the start, and perhaps even to provide training in desktop publishing for the staff involved in producing material for the newsletter. Once produced, copies can be made available for clients to pick up in the waiting room and be included in reminder mailings. A PDF version can be placed on the practice web site.

## Personal Selling

Staff represent the practice in all of their encounters with clients and have plenty of opportunities to promote the services and products that the practice provides. This is not to say that staff should all become salespeople. For most veterinarians, this would go completely against the grain, as their main concern and duty is to ensure the welfare of the animals placed under their care. This does not preclude 'selling', but in a softer form, the aim of which is mutual benefit – for the animal, the owner and the practice.

Nevertheless, all staff should have a sound knowledge of the services and products offered by the practice *and of their benefits*. The 'features–benefits' model should become a natural way of explaining the services and products to clients. Describing the features of each, and following each feature description with an explanation of how this will benefit the pet and owner will help the owner to understand why the service or product will be of use, and is likely to be more convincing than an account of just its features alone. Here is an example of the use of this model where a veterinary nurse is providing information to a client about Frontline Spot On flea treatment:

> We would recommend Frontline Spot On for you to use on Archie. It comes in handy pipettes, which are very easy to use. You simply snip off the tip of the pipette and apply it to your cat's skin at the base of the head and just between the shoulder blades. What's good about it is that your cat will hardly notice the application and you don't have to worry about any side effects. It is very effective against fleas and larvae, but you must remember to apply it every 4 weeks or so. To make sure you don't forget an application, it comes with a set of little labels, which you can fix to your calendar as a reminder of when the next application is due, so that takes care of having to remember.

Staff also need to have complete confidence in the practice and enthusiasm for their jobs. This comes from being valued by their employers through appropriate remuneration for and appreciation of their work. Receptionists are often the lowest paid members of practice staff, even though they are the first point of contact for clients and are instrumental in bringing people in through the practice doors. The selection, training and retention of good receptionists should be a priority for practice owners.

All staff should develop excellent questioning and listening skills – this is key to establishing a client's needs accurately. Asking the right questions and listening to the answers carefully without interrupting and allowing the client to do most of the talking will lead to a better understanding of what is important to the client.

## Direct Marketing

Practice management systems allow reminders, news and information to be sent to clients in a targeted way, either by post, e-mail or text message. Until around 5 years ago, mail was the primary means of sending targeted information, letters and notices about events and promotions. E-mail has now taken over and most clients have an e-mail address to which information can be sent. The advantage of this medium is that it is quick, easy and cost-effective. The disadvantage is that most people will probably ignore such e-mails, as this medium has quickly become overused for marketing. In the UK, it is an offence to send unsolicited marketing e-mails, so practices need to ensure that clients have agreed to receive information by e-mail or text message. In addition, every e-mail should always include an 'unsubscribe' option to enable a client to decide to no longer receive information in this way if they so wish.

While e-mail is an excellent form of communication for small animal practice owners, it may not be quite as effective for farm animal and equine owners who spend a great deal of their time outdoors. Mobile phone text messaging may be the preferred option here.

Generally, response rates to direct marketing are low, but it does allow regular contact with clients, especially with those who only visit the practice once a year. This helps to maintain the practice presence within the client's world, and if the practice can succeed in conveying genuine interest in and knowledge of their animals, clients will appreciate and understand the efforts that are being made.

## Internet and Online Marketing

Now that over 60% of the UK population has access to the Internet and the World Wide Web, it makes sense for all practices to have their own web sites. A web site provides opportunities for gaining new clients, as well as for attracting potential employees. As a minimum, the home page should provide information on how to get in touch, practice opening hours and what to do in an emergency. There are companies that will provide basic web site templates and facilities at a reasonable price, but this does not give the flexibility or freedom of design that practices might want. Specialist web site designers can be expensive, but do allow more say over content, layout and appearance. This is a competitive area and shopping around should enable a practice to find a designer who will provide a good service at a reasonable cost.

Once a web site has been set up, it has to be maintained and updated, which could involve ongoing costs if there is no one in the practice with the necessary skills. Practice web sites now include facilities for booking appointments online and requesting repeat prescriptions, as well as enabling payments to be made.

The advantages of web sites for users are that they are accessible all the year round at a time and place convenient to them. Potentially, a practice web site could be viewed by millions of people. But first, people need to know that it is there, so practices must ensure that they maximize the presence of their web sites on the Internet.

## Public Relations and Publicity

Practices are a part of the communities within which they operate. They also have links with organizations and bodies in the wider external environment, all of which are a part of a practice's daily life. The way in which a practice views its presence in the community and the methods that it uses to develop a relationship with its near and far environments are referred to as public relations. The aim of public relations activities is to raise awareness of the practice in the wider environment, to enhance its reputation and gain support for its work. Public relations activities that are most frequently engaged in by practices include open days and client talks, sponsorship (giving and receiving), press releases and articles in the local press, radio talk shows or phone-ins and participation at veterinary congresses and conferences.

There are no rules that state how much or how little of all of these activities practices should engage in – this is dependent on the practice owners, vets and staff, and how important they consider such activities to be, and which must be done in addition to the daily bread-and-butter work and often require considerable time and effort. There is evidence, however, that public relations (PR) has a positive effect on a number of aspects of practice life and thus cannot be ignored:

- PR can enhance a practice's reputation and raise its profile, which can help to attract good employees and new clients.
- Interesting positive outcome stories about animals and vets heard on the radio or read in the local press have the potential to reach a very large number of people and do result in increased public interest and a desire to purchase.
- Giving talks to local schools and societies increases public goodwill, which in turn increases trust and custom.

At the very least, PR is a way of giving something back to the community from which practices derive their clients and is part of being a 'good citizen'.

Publicity is about disseminating information about services and products without having to pay for it. Unlike an advertisement, however, such information must be highly desirable and newsworthy. If a respected third party writes about the practice, this has high credibility in the eyes of the public, as it is not the practice doing the advertising but someone independent, so is more persuasive than an advertisement. Press releases are usually published free of charge, so there is no cost involved in getting these published in the local papers, even though there is a cost in terms of staff time in writing the press release and then sending it to suitable publications. The downside to this is the loss of control over whether it will be published or not, because if it is not distinctive or newsworthy enough for the publication's readers, then the editor is unlikely to accept it. Stories or articles can potentially be edited and so there is some loss of control over content too.

## Conclusions

A practice's communication mix is crucial to building and maintaining a strong practice–client relationship and is a key part of the relationship-building process. Most practice communications are aimed at gaining and retaining clients and promoting its services and products. Thus, a practice's communication mix is largely synonymous with its promotional mix.

Most practices use a range of communications, but those that are more personalized and targeted to specific client groups, such as personal selling and direct marketing, tend to be more effective than non-personal forms of communication, such as advertising. This is because continued client contact depends on the practice building a relationship with the client longer term, and personalized forms of communication help to do this more effectively.

## References

Jevring-Bäck, C and Bäck, E (2007) *Managing a Veterinary Practice*, 2nd edn. Saunders Elsevier, Philadelphia, Pennsylvania.

Jobber, D. (2001) *Principles and Practice of Marketing*, 3rd edn. McGraw-Hill, Maidenhead, UK.

Page, G. (2009) Does your advertising work? *In Practice* 31, 33–36.

Richardson, M. and Richardson, C. (2010) Newsletters: why they're vital to communication. *The Veterinary Business Journal* No. 97, 16–17.

Sharma, N. and Patterson, P.G. (1999) The impact of communication effectiveness and service quality on relationship commitment in consumer, professional services. *Journal of Services Marketing* 13, 151–170.

## Revision Questions

**1.** What is a practice's 'communication mix' and why is it synonymous with a practice's 'promotional mix'?

**2.** List and explain the components of the 'promotional mix'.

**3.** Explain the advantages and disadvantages of advertising.

**4.** Identify the different forms of communication that your practice engages in and determine how effective these are in attracting new clients.

# 4    The 7 Ps of Marketing Services

Managers involved in marketing services aim to develop an advantage over competitors in seven key areas, known collectively as '*the marketing mix*'. The marketing mix is all about the service and how it is delivered to the client. By analysing each of the elements of the marketing mix, managers will become familiar with all aspects of service delivery and will be able to identify the changes and improvements that need to be made in order to enhance the client experience.

The seven elements of the marketing mix are:

- **Product** – What is the practice offering? What is special or unique about this offering or about the way it is being delivered?
- **Price** – Is the price right both for the client and the practice?
- **Place** – Is the location advantageous? Is there plenty of parking? Is it clearly signposted and inviting to passers-by? Does the web site convey the right image and is it attractive, interesting and optimized for Web browsers?
- **Promotion** – How are clients kept informed about the practice, any new products and services or special offers and promotions?
- **People** – Does the practice employ the right staff? Do they have the necessary technical and interpersonal skills? Do they represent the practice to clients in a manner that is in keeping with the practice ethos?
- **Physical evidence** – Do the 'tangibles', such as the waiting room, consulting rooms, equipment and facilities, meet client expectations?
- **Process** – Are the procedures and processes, as experienced by clients, efficient and effective while at the same time conveying a caring and empathetic approach?

Additional Ps, such as Positioning and Proactivity, have been added over the years to the marketing mix for services, but arguably, these can be viewed as dimensions of the original seven elements.

## Product

To most clients, a first-opinion practice offers a broadly similar core service to any other practice – clients expect their animals to receive the same kind of medical care and drugs, whichever practice they choose to register with. They also take it for granted that all qualified veterinarians and veterinary nurses are competent professionals. Practices do not really have a great deal of scope for differentiation of this core service, other than specialization. They can, however, differentiate themselves in the way in which they provide the services so that clients receive a quality experience which meets their needs and exceeds their expectations. If a practice can do this consistently and reliably, then clients will report high levels of satisfaction.

How do clients determine the quality of a service? Zeithaml and Bitner (2003) cite research carried out by Parasuraman *et al.* (1988), which identifies five specific quality dimensions used by consumers to determine service quality:

1. **Reliability** – The ability to provide positive outcomes consistently and dependably, e.g. clients expect the veterinarian to make a correct diagnosis of their animals' problems and prescribe the correct treatment that will make them better.
2. **Responsiveness** – Readiness to provide a prompt service and assistance at all times, e.g. if clients telephone the practice for advice, they expect to receive it promptly.
3. **Assurance** – Knowledgeable and courteous staff who inspire confidence and trust, e.g. clients want veterinarians to be open and honest with them, to explain their pets' problems in terms they can understand, to clearly outline the available options for treatment and to help them make an informed decision.
4. **Empathy** – A caring, individualized approach, the ability of staff to put themselves in the client's position, e.g. clients expect veterinarians to be

skilled communicators, to really hear their concerns and to demonstrate empathy. Above all, they expect them to care.

**5. Tangibles** – The appearance, atmosphere and professionalism engendered by the physical facilities and personnel, e.g. clients expect the waiting room to be clean and welcoming and the staff to look professional.

Clients will use all of the above dimensions to make a decision about the quality of the service provided and they will build their overall impression from each and every encounter that they have with the practice. However, because clients are not all the same, each will present a unique set of needs and will experience the service in their own unique way. Because of this, achieving consistency in service quality is challenging, and some factors, such as client perceptions, may be beyond the control of the practice.

## Price

The prices a practice charges for its services are determined by a number of factors:

- Practice positioning – is the practice aiming to offer clients a good, basic service or a high-quality service using state-of-the-art equipment and the latest techniques, thus justifying higher prices?
- Species that are treated.
- Geographical location – is the practice rural or urban, inner city or suburb?
- The prices that are charged by direct competitors.
- The level of practice costs that have to be recovered through income.
- The amount of profit the practice owner requires.

All of the above factors, and others specific to the individual practice, will have a direct impact on the pricing strategy that is selected. There are a number of different strategies available, but most practices use a combination of cost-based, competitor and value pricing; these are explained in Chapter 20. Whichever method is chosen, clients expect it to be fair and non-exploitative.

In 2009, the American Animal Hospitals Association (AAHA) commissioned nationwide research funded by Pfizer Animal Health aimed at quantifying practice team improvement of pet care compliance and pet owner adherence to veterinary recommendations. One of the areas investigated was the issue of pet owners' attitudes towards cost and the impact of cost on compliance with and acceptance of veterinarians' recommendations. The results of this research showed that pet owners in the USA generally felt that they were receiving good value from their veterinarians. For these owners, the cost of veterinary care was rarely a factor when choosing a veterinary practice or accepting a veterinarian's recommendations (Albers, 2007). However, the same research also showed that most pet owners had a maximum amount that they were willing to pay for their pet's treatment in any one year. Although this maximum varied between US$500 and US$3000, some 27% of owners indicated that their maximum price was US$500 and 32% indicated that their maximum was US$1000. Clearly, there is a limit to how much pet owners are willing and able to pay, and for a significant number of clients the issue of money will inevitably become a consideration at some point. Because of this, veterinarians should always be prepared to discuss the costs and the various options that are available, which means that they should be thoroughly familiar with the practice's pricing strategy and policies.

Price becomes a definite factor when the perceived quality of the service is poor, though. High prices or price increases will certainly not be tolerated in such cases and clients are very likely to transfer to another practice.

## Place

Veterinary services are usually only available at the practice premises, except in the case of emergencies, so most clients are obliged to bring their animals to the practice. Dog owners may find the process easier than cat owners or owners of other more exotic species, but for all owners and their pets there is a certain amount of inconvenience and stress involved in visiting the practice. Some pets do not travel well, which can be an additional cause of stress. That is why clients prefer a practice that is conveniently located. Location is, in fact, the top determinant of practice choice for prospective clients and the most important factor for practice success (Moreau and Nap, 2010). A convenient location and plentiful parking represents the ideal, although this may not always be achievable, and so practices that are located in less favourable locations need to work harder to gain new clients.

## Promotion

The promotional mix was discussed in Chapter 3. A practice could potentially undertake all of these activities, but without a proper marketing plan, this approach may well be counterproductive. Marketing activities carry a cost and so it is important to ensure that only those activities are undertaken that are consistent with the practice's overall objectives. The marketing plan does not need to be particularly sophisticated. For example, staff could simply brainstorm ideas for specific events or promotions, which could then be evaluated for 'best fit' in terms of what the practice can afford, time of year, client base, staffing and available equipment and facilities. The most appropriate client groups can then be identified to whom the different promotions or activities would be advertised. Following on from this, a plan of action could be devised for the year ahead with timelines and responsibilities assigned.

Promotional activities targeted at specific client groups, and matching the needs and interests of these groups, are more likely to be effective in terms of generating additional revenues. The segments a practice should specifically target are those for which it can provide a competitive product or service. For example, a practice may want to offer acupuncture, but if a direct competitor is already offering this service, then there may be no point going ahead with the idea unless it can be done in a different way or priced more competitively. Of course, it might make sense to go ahead with this service anyway, simply to match the competitor's offerings and thus to remove any advantage that the competitor might have had.

Word-of-mouth recommendation is very important in services. Satisfied and loyal clients will recommend the practice to others. Other strategies, such as talks to community groups, sponsorship of sporting activities or open days, can be very effective in spreading positive word of mouth.

## People

The quality of the employees who provide the service is inseparable from the quality of the service itself (Jobber, 2001). Veterinarians, in particular, play a decisive role in building client trust, which is fundamental to the practice–client relationship. Honesty and openness are the foundations of trust and should be present in all dealings with clients. Clearly, veterinarians need to possess excellent communication skills, especially listening skills, as well as the ability to adapt to different client types and preferences; this may seem a tall order at times, particularly when dealing with difficult clients. Communication skills can be learnt and developed, however, starting at veterinary school where they are taught as an important part of the curriculum. Excellent communication skills are also a fundamental requirement for front-line staff – receptionists and nurses.

It is only possible to employ the right people with the necessary skills if a practice has effective recruitment procedures in place and, subsequently, systems of performance monitoring and control, which ensure that staff know what is expected of them. Training and development are crucial to maintaining skills and ensuring that these are up to date and that they fulfil the needs of both the employer and clients. It is essential to support staff in other ways as well, by providing the equipment and resources they need to do their jobs, showing appreciation for what they do and, of course, offering appropriate remuneration as well as suitable rewards for exceptional performance.

Satisfied employees mean satisfied customers – not in the sense that one causes the other, but rather that the two are interrelated and feed off each other (Zeithaml and Bitner, 2003). This is particularly true within a service business, so employers must treat their staff well.

## Physical Evidence

This element of the marketing mix concerns the 'tangibles' – all the things that clients can see, feel, hear and touch – the environment within which the service is delivered and all the different items associated with it, such as visual displays, leaflets and brochures, uniforms worn by staff, the seating in reception, product displays, etc. The 'tangibles' are inspected by clients who look for clues about the quality of the service which they convey.

Hoffman and Bateson (1997) discuss the impact of visual stimuli, such as size, shape and colour, on client perceptions. Harmony and agreement are associated with plusher, quieter and more formal surroundings with understated colour schemes, while contrast and clash are associated with more exciting, dynamic and informal settings. According to these authors, size matters – the larger the size of the business premises and its physical resources (e.g. spacious waiting room), the more consumers will associate it with importance, power and success. This does not always hold true, however, because some consumers may also view this as impersonal and uncaring.

Two key tangibles that are influential in a potential client's choice of practice are the practice premises and the waiting room, which provide the decisive first impression alongside the reception staff. Prominent, clearly visible, legible and attractive signage, buildings in a good state of repair, a clean and tidy car park, an accessible and welcoming entrance giving the overall impression of a friendly and welcoming practice that takes pride in itself and looks after its environment should be the norm.

Clients should not have to wait longer than 10 minutes to see the veterinarian, but if they do, the time spent waiting should be entertaining and informative. This can be achieved in a variety of ways. A recent modern development is the flat screen TV, displaying a range of informative and entertaining films and images. Useful leaflets and brochures, interesting product displays and seasonal wall displays can be effective in reducing boredom and stress levels. But nothing can substitute for the opportunity to talk informally with a receptionist, veterinary nurse or technician who shows a genuine interest in and enthusiasm for the clients and their animals and who can recommend additional information or give general advice and tips about pet care while the clients wait.

## Process

The procedures which a client experiences, from appointment booking at the beginning, all the way through to payment of the bill by the client and the client taking leave at the end, should be smooth, efficient, consistent and convey a caring, yet professional approach, at all times. Inconsistencies in advice giving, which are a common failure, especially when inexperienced personnel are employed, will not only confuse clients, but may also lead to a lack of faith and trust in the service. New staff should be given a thorough briefing in all of the practice's protocols and procedures before being let loose on clients. Trainees should be supervised at all times by an experienced member of staff and at no time should they be left in a position of having to deal with unfamiliar situations or difficult clients on their own. At the very least, they should know whom to approach for assistance and get the help they need straight away.

Clients are very curious to know what goes on behind the scenes when their animals are admitted for an operation. It makes good sense to show them, either by providing brief tours of the facilities, theatres and wards or by having a photo gallery on the practice web site or a film on the digital screen in the waiting room showing the entire process from admission to discharge, obviously omitting any scenes of animal discomfort or distress. This helps to convey the message that staff are proud of the practice's facilities and are open in everything they do.

Established and efficient communication channels, sharing of information and passing on messages from clients promptly are all essential to the process of providing a good service, as is good teamwork.

When things go wrong, as they inevitably will from time to time, there should be a clear procedure for dealing with client complaints and for putting things right, if possible. There should also be a process for recording and monitoring complaints and learning from them, because client complaints can be a very useful source of information for the practice about areas that it needs to improve.

Clearly, there is a great deal more that could be said about each of these elements of the marketing mix, and it has only been possible to provide a brief overview of the key aspects here. The guidance can be summarized as a set of 'rules for success', as follows:

- Strive to provide a competent, reliable, consistent, responsive and caring service to clients at all times.
- Employ a pricing strategy that fulfils the needs of the business and is fair to clients, and be open with clients about prices, emphasizing the benefits of the products and services provided.
- Target marketing communications and promotions to specific client groups as part of a well-thought-out marketing plan.
- Reward loyal clients who act as ambassadors for the practice by actively promoting it to family, friends and others.
- Good staff are key to the quality of service provision – treat them well!
- Care for the practice environment, both inside and outside, and ensure that the tangible cues of service quality convey the right message.

- Give clients a pleasant, interesting and entertaining waiting room experience and a knowledgeable and enthusiastic member of support staff to talk to while they wait.

## References

Albers, J. (2007) What pet owners really think about cost. *Trends Magazine*, May/June 2007, 45–50. American Animal Hospital Association, Denver, Colorado. Available at: http://trends.aahanet.org/images/CustomContent/PetOwners-Cost.pdf (accessed 3 April 2012).

Hoffman, K.D. and Bateson, J.E.G. (1997) *Essentials of Services Marketing*, 1st edn. The Dryden Press Series in Marketing, Dryden Press, Hinsdale, Chicago, Illinois.

Jobber, D. (2001) *Principles and Practice of Marketing*, 3rd edn. McGraw-Hill, Maidenhead, UK.

Moreau, P. and Nap, R.C. (2010) *Essentials of Veterinary Practice: An Introduction to the Science of Practice Management.* Henston Veterinary Publications, Veterinary Business Development, Peterborough, UK.

Parasuraman, A., Zeithaml, V.A. and Berry, L.L. (1988) Servqual: a multiple-item scale for measuring consumer perceptions of service quality. *Journal of Retailing* 64, 12–40.

Zeithaml, V.A. and Bitner, M.J. (2003) *Services Marketing: Integrating Customer Focus Across the Firm*, 3rd edn. McGraw-Hill Higher Education, New York.

## Revision Questions

1. (a) Carry out a critical assessment of your practice's waiting room, either personally or by conducting a mini survey of client opinions.
   (b) Evaluate your findings and identify the good and the bad points.
   (c) Recommend some changes that would improve the client experience.

2. (a) Familiarize yourself with the practice's complaints procedure, if you have not done so already.
   (b) Find out how many client complaints were received by the practice over the past 12 months and how these were handled.
   (c) Decide whether these complaints were handled well. If not, what would you do differently?

3. (a) If you perform a client-facing role in your practice, list the ways in which you personally contribute to client satisfaction.
   (b) Describe three incidents when you put the clients' needs first before your own.

# 5 The Costs and Benefits of Marketing

## How Much to Spend on Marketing?

At the start of every new financial year, as part of the practice's annual budgeting exercise, managers set aside a marketing budget for promotional and public relations activities. The practice's marketing strategy for the forthcoming year might, for example, include plans to hold an open day, give a series of six client talks and write a regular pet interest column for the local paper, in addition to the usual puppy parties and product sales promotions. Thus, a key question is 'how much to set aside for marketing'? Large organizations spend vast sums of money on marketing, corporate practices can certainly afford more marketing than small, independently owned practices.

There are a number of issues:

**1.** Previous experience can inform the future – a review of the activities undertaken in the last year will give an idea of what worked and what didn't and of the costs involved – at least those costs that can be measured in monetary terms. But next year will certainly not be the same as last year. Next year, additional marketing activity may be required or a new service may need to be promoted more actively, which will result in greater expense, the extent of which may not be known.

**2.** The size of the marketing budget will depend on the other expenses of the practice. More important expenses, such as those that are needed to support the primary function of the practice, will naturally take priority and so, after all of these have been taken into account in the budgeting process, there may not be very much left over for marketing (Forsyth, 2003).

**3.** In order to arrive at a budget, each planned activity could be analysed and costed, and then all the costs could be added together to arrive at a figure. However, it may be difficult to establish the exact costs and so the final figure obtained will be an estimate at best.

The process of budget setting may not be an exact science, but it must, nevertheless, be undertaken, because marketing carries a cost, which must be covered by the increased revenues that it aims to generate.

## The Costs of Marketing – Example

The following example will give an idea of some of the costs involved in marketing activities. Assume that a veterinary practice wishes to hold an open day. Figure 5.1 shows the draft programme for this event, which is planned to take place in June 2012.

### Staff costs

As the programme shows, a great deal of planning is required beforehand if the event is to be a success – at least 2–3 months ahead, perhaps even longer. Support staff time that is spent organizing contributors to the event, producing invitations and arranging publicity should be costed and included in event costs. Time spent planning for an open day is time that is *not* spent earning income. This represents lost income, which should be estimated and also included as an event cost.

Staff involved in running the event on the day may be expected to give of their time freely, but such commitment should not go unrewarded. Staff could be rewarded either in the form of gift vouchers, time off in lieu, flowers or other gifts. The cost of post-event gifts and 'thank-yous' is an event cost.

### Consumables/materials

The cost of consumables that the practice has to pay for, such as pens, badges, brochures, refreshments, prizes and posters, should be added in to the total costs. Food manufacturers and product suppliers are often willing to sponsor specific items, such as prizes, and to provide free samples; this

© C.R. Coates 2012. *Veterinary Practice Management* (C.R. Coates)

**Fig. 5.1.** A. veterinary practice open day draft programme.

Open Day Draft Programme Saturday, 10 June 2012, 12 noon–4 p.m.

| Time | Activity | Personnel | Resources required |
|---|---|---|---|
| 12.00 (noon) | Welcome and opening remarks Welcome to Guest of Honour (GOH) | Principal and GOH | |
| 12.15 p.m. | Practice tours (maximum 20 visitors per tour) | Head nurse | Tour tickets |
| | Every half an hour until 2.45 p.m. | Principal | Gift bags (practice brochure, samples, badges, pens, money-off vouchers) |
| | | Associates × 2 | |
| | Concurrent displays throughout afternoon: | | |
| | • Staff pets in kennelling area | Veterinary nurse | Water bowls, food, litter trays, toys, beds, leads |
| | • Portable ultrasound equipment demonstration | Associate | |
| | • Guide Dogs for the Blind, Hearing Dogs, Pat Dogs, Royal Society for the Prevention of Cruelty to Animals (RSPCA), Royal Society for the Protection of Birds (RSPB), People's Dispensary for Sick Animals (PDSA), Pet Rescue stalls | Receptionist (to liaise) | Tables and coverings × 6–8 plus two smaller tables |
| | • Schools' art competition display | Receptionist | Notice boards |
| | • Raffle (for charity) | Receptionist | Raffle tickets, prizes (discount vouchers?) |
| | • 'Guess the Name of the Pony' competition | Pony owner | Feed, water, whiteboard grid, pens |
| | • Refreshment stall – tea/coffee, biscuits | Practice manager | Table and cloth, urn, tea and coffee, milk, sugar, paper cups and plates, biscuits, price labels, teaspoons |
| | • Ice cream van | | |
| | • Hot dogs and burgers vans | | |
| | • 'Pin the spot-on on the dog' | Veterinary nurse | Large picture of dog and cardboard spot-on pipettes (adhesive) |
| | • 'Knock down the fleas' children's bowling alley | Veterinary nurse | Soft toy 'fleas' and soft balls |
| | • Face painting | Client volunteer | Paints, water, towels, paper towels |
| | • Balloon animals | Client volunteer | Balloons |
| 1.00 p.m. | Dog agility display | Practice manager | Local dog agility team Adjacent field |
| 2.00 p.m. | 'Most Obedient Dog' competition (GOH to judge) | Practice manager | Prizes and rosettes |
| 3.00 p.m. | Grand Prize-giving | Principal and GOH | Adjacent field Public address system |
| 4.00 p.m. | Closing Remarks – Principal and GOH | | *Clean-up – all staff please!* |

**Note**: Security guard to patrol entire area throughout, St John Ambulance to be present – donation??. Risk assess all activities!

helps to reduce these costs, but will not cover everything. The cost of all of these different items should be identified and quantified as accurately as possible. This is easier to do during the planning stage when records of specific orders and purchases are more readily to hand, and a running tally should be kept throughout the planning stage.

### Advertising

Once the programme is agreed and the services of all contributors to the event have been secured, it is necessary to publicize the open day. The cost of producing advertising flyers, leaflets and brochures should be included in the event costs as well as the cost of any direct mailshots and advertisements placed in the local papers, shop windows or any other locations for which there is a charge.

### Overheads

Overheads comprise any proportional establishment costs, such as power, heating and water that would not normally be used if the practice was closed. Establishment costs are difficult to estimate for a specific event such as this, but if the practice premises are kept open especially for the event, then a proportion of the annual costs could be calculated and attributed to the event.

Even though open days are a great day out for clients, their families and friends and are excellent public relations, they are expensive and time-consuming to organize and run. Increased goodwill and an enhanced relationship with the local community may well follow, but clear profit from new business resulting from an open day would need to amount to a considerable sum before the costs are recovered.

A similar costing exercise should be carried out for all marketing activities that are being considered. This will provide a sound basis for budgeting decisions and will help to identify which activities are likely to be the most cost-effective.

### Measuring the Effects of Marketing Activities

Managers should consistently gather data on the effectiveness of marketing campaigns. Without detailed monitoring and analysis of the results of marketing activities, they will only be able to report anecdotal evidence of how effective their open day,

client talk or school visit was in terms of increased sales of products, or numbers of new clients registering with the practice. Most marketing activities carry a cost, but if no income is attributed to marketing efforts, these costs are treated simply as a business expense or loss. This is incorrect, because the fundamental purpose of most marketing activities is to increase practice revenues. If there is no evidence that this is being achieved, why bother with marketing at all?

With the open day example, there are a number of different ways in which its results can be gauged – through discount vouchers or 'free first consult' vouchers handed out on the day and, of course, by continuing to ask new clients where they heard about the practice and why they chose it. Attendees could also be given mini questionnaires to complete about their experience.

Practice computer systems enable a certain amount of analysis, but may not allow continued automatic monitoring of, for example, all clients who had attended a puppy party during the past year and who had remained with the practice over a period of say, the first 3 years, in terms of the number of times they visited the practice or average transaction values per (puppy-owning) client. A separate record of these clients would have to be made and someone would have to take responsibility for interrogating the practice system to ascertain activity on a regular basis. Practices often do not have the staffing resources or the inclination to do this, even though it would only be a question of tracking the activities of a relatively small number of clients. If such monitoring was carried out, however, over a period of up to at least 3 years, this would result in some very useful and revealing hard data, which would help to inform marketing decisions made in the future.

To take the puppy party example further, what information could one expect to obtain from monitoring the activity of puppy owners who had attended a puppy party over a period of, say, the first 3 years of dog ownership, and how useful would this be? Assuming that the dogs remain healthy during this time, there would be data on the following:

- Breed ownership data and ownership duration (for various reasons, some owners will not keep their dogs)
- Attendance at puppy parties and behaviour classes

- Microchipping and any pet passport applications
- Dog grooming appointments kept – if the practice offers this service
- Attendance for annual health checks and booster vaccinations
- Purchases of wormers and flea products
- Purchases of food and toys
- Purchases of dental products
- Attendance at other practice promotional events, such as open days and talks.

Monitoring client activity over a period of time enables a picture of client behaviour to be built up and gaps in service quality to be identified. For example, if 60% of the clients who attended practice puppy parties subsequently left the practice, or if only 10% still remained with the practice 3 years hence, then clearly the practice is doing something wrong and urgently needs to identify what that is in order to prevent new clients leaving.

Monthly flea treatments and 3-monthly worming treatments allow an accurate prediction of client spending on these products over a period of 3 years. If the pattern of spending is consistent, then all is well, but if there are gaps in treatments, or if treatments stop altogether, then it is likely that the client is purchasing these products – and probably other products too – elsewhere. Many practices do not monitor flea and worming treatments consistently and often fail to check that these are up to date when clients visit the practice.

Monitoring allows comparisons to be made between clients who did not attend practice puppy parties and those who did in order to establish whether the puppy parties have any effect on purchasing behaviour or visit frequency. One would expect to see a rise in uptake of products and services immediately after a puppy party by those clients who brought their puppies along. This would then level off, demonstrating that a puppy party does have a temporary positive effect on purchasing behaviour. Proper monitoring would allow this supposition to be proved or disproved, because hard data would be available. In addition to this, the use of client feedback questionnaires would provide additional subjective information about a client's experience and intentions, which could be used alongside objective data, thus building up a richer picture of client behaviour. Each promotional event that this client sample attends could also be monitored for its effects, enabling conclusions to be drawn about the effectiveness of the events and of promotional activities in general.

Unfortunately, such studies are longitudinal in nature and may be way over the top for most small practices. For such a study to be undertaken, it is essential that the selected sample of clients is informed about this research and that each gives permission for it to be carried out, even though it involves no inconvenience to them – otherwise, the practice risks contravening the Data Protection Act 1998, which is covered in Chapter 15.

It is relatively easy to monitor the effects of product promotions through looking at quantities of product sold, before, during and after the promotion. Product promotions, such as 'buy-one-get-one-free' (BOGOF) or reductions in the normal price of a specific product, such as flea treatments, wormers or food, will result in an increase in sales for a period, followed by a levelling off of demand. Offering discounts on products means that the practice's profit is reduced and, therefore, to maintain the level of profit more product needs to be sold.

## Intangible Benefits

From time to time, practices will wish to run specific events, such as free client talks, for which they will happily bear the full cost, without anticipation of any gain, in order to enhance the practice–client relationship and build client goodwill. These benefits are intangible and may not be measured in monetary terms. The manager may well consider that they outweigh the costs incurred if they ultimately result in improved client retention overall, but this is very hard to substantiate, and if the costs are not recovered, reduced profits will result, which will not please the owner. Thus, marketing activities cannot be undertaken simply because they seem to be a good idea at the time, but must ultimately result in real, measurable benefits for the practice.

## Reference

Forsyth, P. (2003) *Marketing Stripped Bare: An Insider's Guide to the Secret Rules*. Kogan Page, London.

## Revision Questions

**1.** Identify a specific marketing activity that your practice engages in regularly.

(a) Analyse this activity in terms of the costs involved versus the benefits gained, as far as you are able to establish these.

(b) Draw conclusions about the cost-effectiveness of the activity.

**2.** Why is it important for practices to monitor the results of their marketing activities?

**3.** Explain how you would monitor the results of a 'buy-one-get-one-free' sales promotion of spot-on flea treatment.

**4.** Your practice wishes to organize a talk for the local community on canine nutrition to be held on a weekday evening outside surgery hours at the local community centre, which hires out rooms at a cost of £80 for 2 hours. A veterinary nurse trained in pet nutrition is willing to give this talk, but it is intended that a veterinarian will also be on hand to provide informal advice and answer any additional client questions. The practice manager has organized tea, coffee and biscuits (at a cost of £26.50) and will use the centre's kitchen facilities for this, which are free of charge. Copies of the practice brochure, relevant leaflets and some free food samples from practice stocks will be handed out. It has been agreed that the nurse and veterinarian will be remunerated for their efforts with a set fee of £25 each. The practice manager has estimated that advertising the event in the local paper will cost £75 for a quarter-page advertisement. Calculate how much this event will cost.

From experience, the practice manager thinks that the event will result in some new clients registering with the practice. The first consultation fee is £30, of which £8 is profit. Calculate how many consultations would be needed to recover the costs of this event.

# SECTION 2
# The Practice–Client Relationship (2): Selecting and Keeping the Right Staff

### Section Objectives

At the end of this section, you should be able to:

- Explain why sound recruitment procedures are essential for practice success.
- Outline a fair and effective procedure for recruiting staff.
- Outline a programme of induction for new staff.
- Understand the importance of staff training and development.
- Explain the purpose of staff appraisal and how this should be conducted.
- Understand what motivates people and the role of performance-related pay, bonuses and rewards as motivators.
- Discuss the concept of leadership and the characteristics of a good leader.

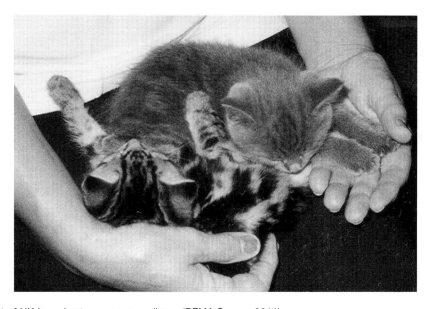

In 2008, 92% of UK-based cats were non-pedigree (PFMA Survey, 2011).

# 6 Recruiting and Selecting Staff

Practice owners would be unable to achieve their goals without the support of their staff. The quality of staff in a veterinary practice determines the quality of the service provided because, as has already been pointed out, service staff represent the service to clients. That is why it is vital to recruit, select and keep the right people. An important aspect of staff retention is the provision of appropriate remuneration for work done, alongside proper appreciation and recognition. This would appear to be common sense, but it is astonishing how many employers still get it wrong.

All businesses, whether large or small, should have an effective human resource management (HRM) programme. Small to medium-sized enterprises, or SMEs (small ≤ 100 people; medium ≥ 100, but < 250 people) are often at a disadvantage compared with larger organizations, primarily because of a lack of resources or of in-house human resources (HR) expertise. Despite this, they should strive to adopt effective HRM practices, specifically in relation to the four main HR functions:

- Recruitment and selection
- Training and development
- Appraisal
- Rewards.

## Why Are Effective Recruitment Procedures Important?

Despite the importance of SMEs to the national economies of the UK, Europe and the USA, there is a paucity of research about how these firms approach HRM tasks. Cassell *et al*. (2002) report that in the USA approximately 99% of employers are small firms. Despite this, little effort has been made to assess the specific challenges that these firms face in the areas of staff recruitment and retention.

A review of the available literature carried out by Cassell *et al*. (2002) reveals that SMEs have a

number of disadvantages compared with larger organizations:

1. The HR expertise and knowledge that are required to manage staff effectively are less likely to be available in house.
2. Staff in SMEs are less likely to have access to a structured programme of training and development.
3. Promotion and progression opportunities within SMEs are likely to be fewer.
4. HRM is unlikely to be linked to strategic objectives in any coherent, structured way.
5. SMEs (including veterinary practices) are constantly emerging and disappearing – this is a continuously shifting scene and so stability and the prognosis for long-term survival are less certain.

These disadvantages mean that HR practices adopted by SMEs are likely to be primarily aimed at satisfying immediate requirements rather than longer term goals. At the same time, the costs of recruiting staff are rising. Leatherbarrow *et al*. (2010) cite a survey carried out by The Chartered Institute of Personnel and Development (CIPD) in 2009 which reports that it costs an average of £4000 per employee to fill a vacancy in the UK. Because recruitment and selection costs are high, it makes sense to ensure that the staff who are offered jobs actually remain with the firm. One way of ensuring this is to have effective recruitment policies and procedures in place.

Another reason for having sound recruitment policies and procedures is the obvious positive influence that these have on the overall financial performance of a business. Huselid (1995) carried out a survey of nearly 1000 US firms to determine whether '*high performance HR practices*' had an impact on a business's financial performance. The HR practices considered included comprehensive employee recruitment and selection procedures, incentive schemes, extensive employee training and development, and employee participation in decision making. Huselid found that HR practices did have a statistically significant impact on employee productivity and on the short- and long-term financial performance of a business. Hiltrop (1996), although sceptical about the availability of 'real' evidence that HRM policies and practices do actually improve the financial performance of a business, was obliged to concede that there is growing evidence that such policies and practices have a positive influence on employees and actually motivate them to exhibit behaviours and attitudes that are conducive to improving their organization's competitiveness.

So it makes sound business sense to apply effective HR policies and procedures. Not only this, but also the overall impact on staff morale will be positive, because effective HRM is concerned not only with recruitment and selection, but also with employees' professional needs during the entire time that they spend with the organization.

## Recruitment

### The job description

The procedures that are described in this and subsequent chapters in this section are suitable for implementation by SMEs. HRM is a complex area of management, so from time to time expert advice will need to be sought by those responsible for staffing and this must be borne in mind. Another important point to note is that no matter how effective the procedures and policies are, positive outcomes cannot always be guaranteed and sometimes the match between an individual and the organization may turn out to be not as ideal as originally thought.

Job vacancies can arise in a number of different ways:

- Normal staff dynamics – a member of staff may leave, another may go on maternity leave and yet another may be off work because of long-term illness, etc.
- Business expansion and growth – the practice may be expanding and may need to take on additional staff.
- Future planning – business strategies may require additional staff or may bring with them changes to the existing staffing structure that result in a vacancy.

Whenever a vacancy arises, for whatever reason, this is an opportunity to review existing staffing levels as well as the existing skills and to identify where there are gaps that need to be filled. This should be done as a routine practice, because the job that has been vacated may not need to remain exactly the same as before. It could be that the duties the postholder performed may be readily apportioned among existing staff, thus making room for a new post that fits practice needs and its future plans much better.

Once a decision to recruit externally has been made, however, it is essential to produce a written *job description* that results from a careful analysis of the post and the duties involved. A job description can serve several different purposes:

- It is the primary source of information about the job for potential applicants.
- It is the primary source of information about the job for existing staff.
- It is the basis upon which the employer sets performance targets and goals for the job-holder.
- It is the jobholder's point of reference about his/her job.
- It can form the basis for discussions at a staff appraisal meeting.
- It can help to prevent misunderstandings about duties and responsibilities.

For these reasons, job descriptions are crucial documents, and should be prepared with care and attention to detail.

All staff who will be working with the postholder, either as fellow team members or in a supervisory capacity, should have input into the job description, as they are the ones who are most familiar with the duties and tasks to be carried out. A job description describes the job itself in detail – the job title, place of work, job purpose, reporting lines, main duties and responsibilities, scope of the post, and provisions for training and development and career progression. Background information about the practice can also be included, in greater detail than appears on the practice web site, to enable potential applicants to build up an accurate picture of the practice and of how the job fits within it. An example of a job description for a veterinary nurse is given in Fig. 6.1. A job description template can be found in Section 6.

'A Veterinary Practice'
Address
Tel:
E-mail:
Web site:

**Veterinary Nurse**
**Job Description**

**Practice Information**

A Veterinary Practice, now in its fifth year of operation, is a modern and rapidly expanding small animal practice in the heart of the Cotswolds. The practice's two partners are supported by three veterinary assistants, 12 qualified VNs and 3 animal care technicians. There are four part-time receptionists and a practice manager supported by two administrative staff employed in the practice office. Staff enjoy the use of modern facilities and equipment with state-of-the-art digital X-ray, ultrasonography and endoscopy facilities. There are three operating theatres, two procedures rooms, a dedicated X-ray suite, a scrub-up area and large wash-up and sterilization area complete with a 20 cubic feet autoclave. The practice has 8000 registered clients and an annual turnover of approximately £1.75 million. The practice prides itself on its close relationship with the local community and maintains this by organizing and participating in several key local events and fund-raising activities throughout the year. Once a year in the summer staff enjoy a day away from the practice, which is spent on team-building activities and developing the practice strategy for the year ahead. The awayday culminates in a practice dinner and prize-giving. The practice is an equal opportunities employer dedicated to developing its staff through the provision of appropriate training and development opportunities.

**Overall Purpose of the Job**

This post is key to the efficient functioning of the practice. Its purpose is to provide veterinary nursing support to the veterinarians both during consultations and when undertaking clinical procedures, and to ensure the smooth functioning of the practice as a whole by following the correct practice protocols and procedures in a timely and efficient manner.

**Location**

The post is located at <address>.

**Working Hours**

The postholder will work 8 hours per day on a rota basis. Starting and finishing times will vary, depending on the rota. There will be a one-hour unpaid break during the working day. Staff working a single shift of 6 or more hours' duration are entitled to a 20 minute rest break. The postholder will also be required to work 4 consecutive nights every 10 weeks, as part of the out-of-hours rota. The salary for out-of-hours work is paid at twice the normal rate.

**Salary Range**

Starting salary will be within the range £20,000–£25,000 negotiable, depending on skills and experience.

**Reporting Lines**

The post reports to the Head Nurse and will have supervisory responsibility for the work of the practice's two animal care assistants.

**Duties**

1. Assisting the consulting and surgical veterinarians with clinical procedures, as per the duty rota.
2. Providing pre- and post-operative care to patients, as required by the veterinary surgeon in charge of the case.
3. Maintaining the cleanliness and hygiene of the surgical suite, wards, consulting rooms and reception area in collaboration with the other practice nurses.
4. Ensuring that the consulting room cupboards and drawers are kept fully stocked and tidy.

**Fig. 6.1.** A job description for a Veterinary Nurse.

*Continued*

**5.** Taking X-rays, blood and urine samples, as instructed, and dealing with these in accordance with practice protocols.

**6.** Supervising the work of the animal care assistants, allocating work, devising rotas and providing on-the-job training.

**7.** Occasional reception work (mainly to cover for sickness absences) involving issuing drugs and medicines to clients and explaining how these should be administered, billing correctly for work done, taking payments and booking appointments using RX Works, the practice management system.

**8.** Ordering drugs, medicines and consumables to restock the practice pharmacy, ensuring adequate stock levels and good stock management at all times.

**9.** Maintaining accurate patient records detailing all treatments applied, client communications and client/patient information provided.

**10.** Maintaining a good working relationship with all team members.

**11.** Carrying out any other reasonable duties as assigned by the Head Nurse.

### Scope of the Job

The postholder will have the authority to place orders with suppliers up to a maximum value of £500 per order. Responsibility for the controlled drugs cupboard and adherence to proper procedures for ordering, handling, storage and disposal of controlled drugs lie within the scope of this post.

### Development and Promotion Opportunities

The practice offers a CPD allowance of £450 p.a. to all veterinary nurses towards training costs. Training needs are reviewed annually as part of the staff appraisal process. Depending on skills, experience and current performance, an opportunity for promotion to Deputy Head Nurse or Head Nurse will be offered should either of these posts fall vacant.

### Specific Training Provided

Training is provided in the use of the RX Works practice management system, as required. A health and safety induction is given within the first week of starting work and full familiarization with practice policies, protocols and procedures is arranged as part of the practice's formal induction procedures. On-the-job training is provided on an ad hoc basis, to fill any skills gaps that might arise.

CPD, continuing professional development.

**Fig. 6.1.** Continued.

Job descriptions are official documents, which should be kept on file as part of the recruitment and selection records for a post, and which should be made available to applicants. It is important to realize that jobs tend to change over time and so a job description drawn up at the start of a post may no longer be relevant. It is essential to amend the job descriptions of existing staff periodically to include any significant changes of duties and responsibilities that take place so that they correctly reflect the current situation. The staff appraisal process offers an opportunity to review job descriptions, and this process is described in Chapter 8.

### The person specification

Once the job description has been finalized, the next step in the recruitment process is to draw up a person specification. A person specification is a description of the *ideal* person for the job and will include details about the essential qualifications, skills, experience and personal qualities that the ideal postholder will possess. A person specification will include both essential and desirable-but-not-essential criteria. The inclusion of both types of criteria will encourage a wider range of applicants to apply for the post and will prevent undue limitations being imposed by adhering to strict criteria in which there is no flexibility. It is important to list criteria that can actually be measured and assessed and to decide what measures should be used. The person specification that accompanies the Veterinary Nurse job description given in Fig. 6.1 is shown in Fig. 6.2. A template for a person specification is provided in Section 6.

A Veterinary Practice
Address
Tel:
E-mail:
Web site:

**Veterinary Nurse
Person Specification**

| | **Essential** | **Desirable** |
|---|---|---|
| **1. Academic Qualifications** | • Minimum of 5 GCSEs at Grade C or above, including Science, Maths and English<br>• RCVS Listed Veterinary Nursing Qualification | • Diploma in Advanced Surgical Nursing<br>• A1 Assessors Award |
| **2. Knowledge** | • Knowledge of current and new pre- and post-operative animal care techniques and protocols<br>• Familiar with latest anaesthetic induction and monitoring procedures<br>• Sound knowledge of commonly used drugs and medicines and their administration, handling and safe storage<br>• Up-to-date knowledge of theatre cleaning and disinfection protocols<br>• Up-to-date knowledge of X-ray protocols and radiation safety procedures<br>• Up-to-date knowledge of health and safety procedures when working in a clinical environment | • Working knowledge of RX Works practice management system<br>• Familiar with latest developments in the field of veterinary medicine and veterinary nursing research |
| **3. Skills** | • Proven competence and skill in carrying out veterinary nursing duties, as listed in the job description<br>• Confidence and experience in effective handling and restraint of animals | • Experience of advanced surgical nursing techniques |
| **4. Experience** | • Post-qualification veterinary nursing experience<br>• Experience of front-line reception work | • Pharmacy management experience<br>• ICU experience |
| **5. Supervisory Experience** | • Experience of providing training in basic animal care skills and devising training schedules for junior staff | • Experience of devising and implementing training schedules for animal care technicians |
| **6. Communication Skills** | • Excellent interpersonal skills<br>• Ability to communicate effectively with clients<br>• Ability to work well alone or as part of a team | • Presentation skills developed through giving client talks and participating in other client educational events |
| **7. Personal Attributes** | • Flexible and adaptable<br>• Self-motivated<br>• Able to take the initiative<br>• Ability to work efficiently under pressure | • Able to handle emergencies calmly and competently |
| **8. Other Skills Required** | • Holder of clean driving licence | • Licensed to drive a van |
| ICU, intensive care unit; RCVS, Royal College of Veterinary Surgeons. | | |

**Fig. 6.2.** A person specification for the post of Veterinary Nurse.

## Advertising the post

The next step in the recruitment process is to advertise the job in a place where suitable candidates are likely to spot it. For professions, such as veterinary medicine, there are usually professional journals and publications specific to the profession. In the UK, the two key publications for advertising jobs are the *Veterinary Record* (the weekly journal of the veterinary profession) and the *Veterinary Times* (also a weekly publication). Both are widely distributed to all veterinarians and veterinary practices, which means very widespread coverage. Employers who wish to advertise outside the profession have at their disposal the local press and should select one or two good publications. Some employers may also wish to contact their local Job Centre Plus with details of the vacancy. For key positions, however, it may be necessary to recruit the services of a specialist recruitment consultant who specializes in veterinary appointments here in the UK. Although expensive, such specialist recruiters have at their disposal greater resources than do many veterinary practices, together with the additional advantage of expert knowledge of effective recruitment and selection procedures. Whether a practice chooses to go it alone or hire the services of a recruitment agency depends largely on the available expertise within the practice, past recruitment success and the funds that are available for recruitment.

When drawing up a job advertisement, the following content is essential:

- Practice logo and name
- Job title
- Job location
- Brief statement of the purpose of the job/synopsis of job content
- How to apply – curriculum vitae (CV) or application form
- Contact name and number/e-mail address or web site URL for enquiries and/or to download an application form
- Deadline date for applications.

It is debatable whether to include salary information in the advertisement or not. Veterinary advertisers tend not to do so because they are very secretive about pay, but it is useful for potential applicants to include at least a salary range.

It is essential to ensure that any content is non-discriminatory, which means that there should be no statements in the advertisement that would directly or indirectly prevent some people applying for the post because of specific racial, gender or other personal characteristics. Job advertisements will often contain statements designed to encourage applications from under-represented groups, for example '*The Pandar Veterinary Group is an equal opportunities employer*'. However, the use of such statements is now becoming less common because it is understood that all employers are now 'equal opportunities' employers. Students are encouraged to familiarize themselves with the provisions of the Equality Act 2010, which consolidates all anti-discrimination legislation in the UK.

Here are two examples of typical job advertisements which could appear in the *Veterinary Times* – one for a veterinary nurse and the other for a veterinary surgeon:

---

(No logo)
**Anytown Veterinary Centre**
**Anytown, Yorkshire**

Following internal promotion, we are looking for an enthusiastic and highly motivated RVN to join our team of 2 vets, 4 nurses and 3 receptionists. We are a friendly, modern and well-equipped small animal practice. Competitive salary, CPD encouraged and funded. 1-in-4 Saturdays (time off in lieu) and no emergency OOH.

For further information, please contact Peggy White, Practice Manager, Anytown Veterinary Centre, Anytown, Yorkshire, YO2 4BZ, tel. 01534 867928 or e-mail peggy@anytownvets.co.uk

---

**Logo**
**A Veterinary Group**

**Veterinary Surgeon – Preston**

We have an opportunity for an experienced small animal practitioner to join our group of progressive surgeries. We are well established in Preston, Bolton and Blackburn and are looking for a veterinary surgeon to take sole charge of our Preston surgery. The ideal candidate will be able to effectively manage a small team of nurses and receptionists and possess a good track record in providing high quality care to patients and excellent customer service to their owners. We can offer:

*Access to a range of modern, quality diagnostic equipment
*A generous CPD allowance
*Competitive salary and generous holidays
*The chance to be part of a supportive and forward-thinking team

Send CV and covering letter to the principal, Simon Easter, E-mail
seaster@tweentownvets.co.uk

Unfortunately, because of space limitations, advertisements tend to impart limited useful information. The first example merely invites enquiries and so clearly the practice is taking a fairly leisurely approach to recruiting a nurse. Presumably, the practice manager has plenty of time on their hands to field telephone enquiries and e-mails even before the recruitment process begins properly. Neither advertisement offers any information about salary range, which would be useful for potential applicants, especially for the second post, which carries with it considerable responsibility. Neither gives a deadline date for applications to be received, suggesting that in both instances potential applicants might have a long wait before they hear anything. The first advertisement says very little about the type of candidate being sought. In fact there is little information in the advertisement altogether, its purpose being mainly to flag up that there is a job and to invite enquiries. The second advertisement provides more information about the role that the postholder will be required to fulfil and the amount of experience being sought. The practice principal, however, is happy to accept CVs with a covering letter and so may, conceivably, be swayed by the quality of the CV submitted and may well miss important and relevant information.

Neither advertisement gives any reason why applicants should choose to apply to these practices rather than elsewhere – they sell themselves very poorly indeed with meaningless and worn out phrases such as 'friendly', 'modern' or 'forward-thinking'. That is the nature of many such job advertisements, so it is incumbent upon the applicants to seek out further information before applying. This can be done in a number of different ways – by telephoning or e-mailing the practice and requesting a copy of the job description and person specification (not all practices will have such documents, so applicants should beware), by asking to speak informally to the line manager, principal or practice manager and/or presenting them with a list of questions, or by asking for a face-to-face meeting and an informal visit. Well-run practices who value their staff will encourage visits and will be happy to provide as much information about the post as is required.

## Application Form or Curriculum Vitae?

CVs vary greatly in format. Reading and sorting through them can be time-consuming and there is a risk that decisions may be made based on how professional a CV looks rather than on its content. Also, some important information may be missing from CVs, thus necessitating extra effort to obtain it. Application forms, in contrast, provide a standardized format for all applicants to use. When designing the form, an employer can ensure that all the important questions are included and that the form fits the format of the job description, thereby making shortlisting much easier. As the recruitment and selection process should be applied equally to all applicants, application forms help to maintain a consistency of approach.

The arrival of application forms into a practice following advertising of the post marks the end of the recruitment process and the start of the selection process.

## Selection

### Shortlisting applicants

All application forms should be recorded as soon as they arrive and a list of all applicants should be drawn up. The forms will then undergo several stages of scrutiny, the first one aimed at rejecting all the applicants who most obviously do not fit the requirements of the job description or do not match the person specification. This initial screening can be carried out by the practice manager or person responsible for human resources in a practice. A shortlisting form is then drawn up that lists the remaining applicants. Their applications are scrutinized carefully again by a panel possibly comprising the practice principal, line manager, practice manager (if there is one) or other appropriately qualified member of staff. The shortlisting panel will usually also carry out the interviews. The panel will aim to reduce the applications down to a suitable number to invite for interview – usually six or seven applicants. A copy of an application shortlisting form is given in Section 6. This form provides space to indicate whether to reject an applicant or whether to invite for interview. The reasons for rejecting an application are listed on the form as an aide-memoire for the shortlisting panel, although they are free to add their own reasons if they wish. The shortlisting form is a formal document and should be kept on file as part of the paperwork pertaining to that particular appointment. All paperwork for the shortlisted applicants should be kept for at least 6 months after a vacancy has been filled.

Once the panel has decided who to invite for interview, all candidates will be informed in writing about the decision. A practice should endeavour to project the right image to the public at all times. This includes job application rejection letters, which should provide as much specific detail as possible about the reasons for rejection.

The shortlisting process is a highly subjective one, but the level of subjectivity is reduced by having more than one person carry out the shortlisting. Subjectivity is also reduced by having a standard procedure, which is followed for all vacancies and, particularly, by ensuring that individuals involved in staff selection undergo fair and effective recruitment training. Even though this training may be expensive, it is money well spent, as it will help to prevent expensive selection errors occurring, errors that could, potentially, lead to litigation.

### Preparing to interview

Although a range of different selection methods is available to employers, the interview is still the most frequently used method in veterinary practices in the UK, despite the fact that research evidence exists which demonstrates that interviews are not a reliable method of candidate selection. Kirkwood and Ralston (1999) point out some of the shortcomings of interviews:

- There is a power imbalance in an interview situation which favours the interviewer and automatically places the interviewee at a disadvantage, and this can act as a barrier for the interviewee.
- Inexperienced interviewers may not be skilled enough to ask the sorts of questions that would generate meaningful information about the candidates.
- From the interviewee's point of view, the interview is a very poor method of finding out about the organization, as interviewees will try to avoid asking 'me-oriented' questions and instead will ask questions that interviewers expect to hear.
- Interviewees put on a 'performance' at an interview which is geared towards impressing the panel and which may not reflect their actual performance in the job.

Nevertheless, the combination of a lack of financial and time resources in veterinary practice necessitates the use of this method of selection although, increasingly, the interview is being supplemented by ability tests and work sampling, which are considered to be more reliable methods of assessing the potential to perform a job.

Before the interview, preparatory work needs to be undertaken. A suitable day and date needs to be set to ensure that all the panel members are available and that the candidates receive sufficient notice of the interview date and time. Candidates should be sent all relevant information, together with clear instructions about whom to report to on arrival. This can be done by e-mail or by post, whichever is the preferred method. E-mail provides a very fast, convenient and economical way of communicating and it does enable candidates to acknowledge receipt of information and confirm attendance quickly and conveniently as well. However, it must be borne in mind that e-mail is not a secure medium and there is a serious risk of confidentiality breaches occurring. Any personal or private information should not be sent by e-mail.

Once all the candidates have been notified and have confirmed attendance, and the panel has been informed, other staff in the practice should also be notified, particularly the receptionists. Receptionists should be given instructions about greeting candidates, directing them and contacting the staff in charge.

### The interview

The interview panel will consist of at least two people, and preferably three or four. The person in charge of organizing the interviews will ensure that the panel members read the job description and person specification, the application forms and any supporting material before the interviews.

The panel should meet half an hour before the start of interviews to agree on the structure of the interview and the questions that will be asked. One member of the panel will take on the role of 'chair' and timekeeper and will manage the entire process. To share the workload, each panel member could be asked to focus on one or two specific criteria and to ask questions about these. Care should be taken to cover all the key requirements for the post. All candidates should be asked the same questions, but questioning should remain flexible to enable a deeper exploration of topics, if necessary. Campion *et al.* (1997) advise the use of situational and behavioural type questions, for example, asking what the candidate would do in specific situations or in a specific scenario, or asking about past behaviour in specific situations. Asking candidates for their opinions or asking questions that require self-evaluation is not recommended, as candidates will be tempted to provide answers they think the panel want to hear, which may not reflect what they really think or believe.

The interview will normally follow a set structure, as follows:

1. The chair welcomes the interviewee, introduces the panel and describes how the interview will be conducted, allowing the interviewee to ask for clarification, if necessary. The chair puts the interviewee at ease and ensures that he/she is comfortable with the proposed structure.

2. Panel members then take it in turns to ask their questions, ensuring that the interviewee does most of the talking and utilizing good questioning and listening skills. The chair monitors the process and ensures good timekeeping.

3. The chair then asks the candidate if he/she has any questions and allows time for these to be answered fully.

4. The chair concludes the interview by thanking the interviewee for attending and explaining the next stage of the process, including the making of the necessary checks, information on when a decision will be made and how this will be communicated to the interviewee.

Assessment of candidates should be systematic and in accordance with an agreed scoring system. To aid this process, a candidate interview assessment form could be used by panel members; this should contain at least four key criteria with a score for each one, to reflect their relative importance. Candidate scores are added together to give a total overall score. The panel members' scores can then be transferred to a report form held by the chairperson, which summarizes all the scores and indicates the candidate with the highest score. Panel members will discuss the candidates' interview performance in light of these scores and will recommend the appointment of one of the interviewees, with a reserve also selected in the event that the chosen candidate refuses the offer of the job.

Before offering a candidate the job, some checks will need to be carried out. Some of these checks are essential by law, such as the verification of identity and of the right to work in the UK. Additional checks, such as of professional qualifications, RCVS membership and references will also be necessary. Candidates can legitimately be asked to bring their passports or photo driving licences to interview, as well as proof of qualifications, so that these can be checked and copied for the files at that stage. References are normally taken up after the interview. The value of references is now mostly limited to confirming the facts of a previous position held, as most employers will prefer to limit themselves to facts that can be verified and will avoid expressing opinions about ex-employees, for obvious reasons.

### The employment contract

Once the necessary checks have been completed satisfactorily, all the interviewees should be notified of the outcome. This should ideally be done in person by the practice principal or practice manager by telephone, and then followed up in writing. The successful candidate will be offered the post and asked if they would like to accept. An offer and an acceptance of a post creates a legally binding contract, so there could be grounds for litigation if a candidate accepts the offer of a job and the practice proceeds on this basis, only for the candidate to subsequently withdraw from the position at a later stage.

It is a legal requirement in the UK that all employees receive a written statement of the main terms and conditions of employment within 8 weeks of starting work (Employment Rights Act 1996). This is not the contract of employment, but could be included in a contract, if required. Such a statement should include the following information by law:

- Names and addresses of employer and employee
- Place of work
- Job title
- Working hours
- Arrangements for payment of salary
- Holiday entitlement
- Pension entitlement
- Details of disciplinary and grievance procedures
- Amount of notice to be given and received on termination of employment
- Sickness and sick pay arrangements.

In addition to this statement, practices should issue all new employees with a written contract of employment before they start work. Both parties should agree to the contract and sign it. Each party should retain a copy.

Contracts vary as to content, but will generally contain details of the following, *in addition* to the statement of the main terms and conditions:

- Details of key practice HR policies, e.g. training and development, appraisals, pay rises, payment of bonuses, if applicable
- Participation in practice rotas
- OOH (out of hours) policy and participation

- Professional behaviour standards expected of employee
- Accommodation – if this is provided – and what the employee's obligations are in relation to this accommodation
- Insurances
- Benefits
- CPD (continuing professional development)
- Health and safety procedures and training provided
- Dress code
- Staff facilities
- Termination of employment – notice periods
- Prospects for future development and progression.

It is advisable to employ the services of a solicitor or employment lawyer when drawing up contracts for the first time to ensure that the terminology and contents are appropriate and legal.

Once contracts have been signed and exchanged and a start date agreed, the practice will make preparations to welcome its new member of staff.

### References

Campion, M.A., Palmer, D.K. and Campion, J.E. (1997) A review of structure in the selection interview. *Personnel Psychology* 50, 655–704.

Cassell, C., Nadin, S., Gray, M. and Clegg, C. (2002) Exploring human resource management practices in small and medium sized enterprises. *Personnel Review* 31, 671–692.

Hiltrop, J.-M. (1996) The impact of human resource management on organisational performance: theory and research. *European Management Journal* 14, 628–637.

Huselid, M.A. (1995) The impact of human resource management practices on turnover, productivity and corporate financial performance. *The Academy of Management Journal* 38, 635–672.

Kirkwood, W.G. and Ralston, S.M. (1999) Inviting meaningful applicant performances in employment interviews. *Journal of Business Communication* 36, 55–76.

Leatherbarrow, C., Fletcher, J. and Currie, D. (2010) Recruitment. In: Leatherbarrow, C. and Fletcher, J. (eds) *Introduction to Human Resource Management: A Guide to HR in Practice*. The Chartered Institute of Personnel and Development, London, pp. 119–136.

### Revision Questions

**1.** Distinguish between a job description and a person specification and explain the purpose of these two documents.

**2.** Rewrite the two job advertisements given in this chapter to ensure that all the essential information is included. In doing so, be more specific about the individual qualities and key experience and skills being sought.

**3.** How can subjectivity be minimized when short-listing applicants for interview?

**4.** If you had applied for a job and were offered an interview, how would you prepare for this?

**5.** What are the shortcomings of interviews as a candidate selection method and how can these shortcomings be minimized?

**6.** Why is it important to have a standardized recruitment procedure supported by standardized documentation?

**7.** (a) Assess the cost of recruiting a member of staff – in terms of staff time and physical and financial resources.

(b) Draw conclusions from your assessment.

# 7 Induction, Staff Training and Development

Every new employee will experience a degree of anxiety about starting a new job and will wonder whether they will be able to settle in quickly and do the job well. Before starting work, a new employee should be told where and to whom to report. All staff should be informed about their new member and should be ready to welcome them and provide support and information, as required. Office space (including a computer and any other office equipment) should be made available and ready, as well as a secure place where personal belongings can be left. This should all be done before the employee's first day. Any overalls, uniforms and other protective clothing and footwear needed for the job (if supplied by the employer) should also be obtained. If the employee will be required to carry an identity badge and access keys to certain areas or the dangerous drugs cupboard, these should be ordered in time so that they can be handed out on the first day. All of these things are important and contribute to a new employee feeling welcome and valued. They may not increase that employee's well-being in themselves, but their absence will certainly increase anxiety and feelings of dissatisfaction.

Shilcock (2011) advises that new employees should not be expected to work on their first day and, ideally, that there should be a period of overlap between the old employee leaving and the new employee starting. If this overlap is not possible, extra cover may need to be brought in for at least the first few days.

## 'Buddy'

Whether the new employee is a veterinarian, veterinary nurse or animal care assistant, they should be assigned a 'buddy' or 'mentor' whose role is to look after them during the first few weeks. The 'buddy' would ideally be a colleague of the same or similar grade and job role whom the new employee can shadow and approach for guidance on a range of day-to-day issues. That person does not need to be available all the time, but should be familiar with the needs of new employees and be able to show them where everything is and explain the routines and culture of the practice to them. The person should also be able to introduce the new employee informally to other members of staff and colleagues. Employers often underestimate the amount of knowledge that is needed to do a job and wrongly assume that everything can be covered by the staff handbook or induction checklist. There is also the assumption that people can simply step into a post because they are professionally qualified, but practices do differ in the ways they do things and it is these differences and new ways of working that have to be learnt. A 'buddy' is invaluable for this purpose.

## Induction Checklist

Practices should ensure that they have a consistent and well-designed induction training programme in place for all new employees. Alongside the informal 'buddy' scheme, there should also be a formal, timetabled induction programme, for which the new employee's line manager is responsible. The line manager's role is to ensure that the induction programme is completed in a timely fashion and signed off. Health and safety training must be completed by law as soon as possible after the new employee starts work, and requires both the employer and the employee to sign that it has been satisfactorily completed. Other training can be delivered in a variety of ways – either in written form, online or in person by suitable members of staff, so long as this is done in an organized fashion. A checklist can be helpful both for the new employee and the line manager. This allows tracking of the training provided and completed, and regular progress reviews. An example of such a checklist is given in Section 6. It is advisable not to

© C.R. Coates 2012. *Veterinary Practice Management* (C.R. Coates)

overload the new employee with information at the start, but to gradually introduce information over a period of a week to 2 weeks, depending on the quantity of information that needs to be imparted and the complexity of the job and work environment. This should be prioritized to enable the employee to become productive in the new job as quickly as possible.

## Practice Handbook

The staff handbook contains copies of all the protocols and procedures that apply, together with copies of practice policy documents. However, it is only going to be of use if it is kept up to date and complete, so someone needs to take responsibility for this and it is usually the practice manager. The handbook does not need to be provided in paper-based form. An online handbook is much easier to keep updated. New employees will need time to familiarize themselves with the handbook's contents, so 'reading time' should be built into the induction timetable. The new employee should be asked to sign a form confirming that he/she has read and understood the handbook.

## Progress Reviews

It is important for the line manager to review a new employee's progress at frequent intervals at the start of employment – weekly for the first few weeks, then at the end of the first month and subsequently at 3 and 6 months. The line manager will also monitor the effectiveness of the induction process and will make any necessary changes in response to employee feedback.

## Needs of Specific Types of Worker

Some new workers may require additional support at the start.

## Young workers

School leavers may have never seen the inside of a veterinary practice before. Health and safety are particularly important here and in the UK there are laws protecting workers between the ages of 16 and 18 (classed as 'young workers') in the workplace. The main provisions of these laws are as follows:

- Young workers are not permitted to work more than 40 hours per week.
- If they work for more than 4.5 hours, they are entitled to a 30 minute rest break, which must be taken in the middle of the work period.
- They are entitled to 12 hours rest in every 24 hour period and must take 2 days off each week, taken together with no working in between.
- Young workers generally cannot work between 10.00 p.m. and 6.00 a.m. (or 11.00 p.m. and 7.00 a.m., by agreement), but there are exceptions to this rule depending on the type of occupation and whether night-time work is crucial to the job.
- A risk assessment must be carried out before a young person starts work and the results notified to them together with details of any measures taken to eliminate the hazards and minimize risks as far as possible.
- Young persons are not permitted to do work that might expose them to radiation or extremes of noise, heat or vibration, or work that requires physical effort beyond their capabilities, e.g. heavy lifting.
- Full training must be provided and the employer must ensure that young people can do the work competently and safely.
- Young workers should be given adequate supervision and may require closer and more direct supervision than adult workers.

## Returners to work

People returning to work after a long period of absence will most likely be out of touch with the changes and developments that have taken place while they were away. The practice may have acquired new equipment or new computer software, for which returners will need training to become familiar with. Induction programmes for such employees need to take these issues into account and allow extra settling-in time and the provision of specific training to bring their skills up to date.

## Disabled workers

The key to ensuring that disabled workers fit in well is to preplan and prepare. Depending on the nature of the disabled workers' specific needs, adjustments to premises, workstations and equipment may be required. Expert advice may need to be sought in order to ensure that all suitable provisions are in place. In the UK, advice is available to employers from the Department for Work and Pensions or Business Link.

## Trainees

Newly qualified veterinarians completing the Professional Development Phase, trainee veterinary nurses or animal care assistants working towards gaining their professional qualifications will want reassurance that the practice can help them to fulfil all the requirements of their qualifications. They will need to complete learning logs and prepare for and sit examinations. It is essential that such staff have good supervision, an agreed schedule of work and regular progress reviews, as well as a commitment from the management team to their success.

## Staff Training and Development

### Why develop staff?

Induction training marks the beginning of ongoing training and development, which should be provided for all staff by every organization, no matter how small. This may seem like a tough demand considering the potentially high costs of training and development and the limited resources available, but research has shown that such investment does pay for itself in terms of:

- Improved staff morale and productivity
- Reduction in staff turnover
- Increased revenues
- Improved chances of business success
- Business growth and development (Business Link, 2011).

The fundamental rationale for staff training and development is quite simple – staff need to be able to deliver the results that managers want and must actually want to do so. The training and development provided ensure that the skills are there to achieve the first objective, while staff motivation contributes to the achievement of the second (Forsyth, 2001).

### The distinction between 'training' and 'development'

It is important to be clear about the distinction between training and development. Cole (2004) defines training as preparation for a specific occupation or job role. Training, according to Cole, is job oriented rather than person oriented. Development, in contrast, is about the person and is more career oriented. While training largely concerns itself with satisfying immediate needs, development takes a broader view of the employee and his/her potential for the future. Forsyth (2001) supports this view by making a similar distinction. He views training principally as a method of ensuring that immediate skills gaps are filled and development as contributing to the longer term effectiveness of both the organization and the individual. Training can contribute to an individual's development, but development is much more than just training.

### Identifying training needs

Training needs can arise in a variety of different ways:

- The practice may acquire some new equipment which staff need to learn how to use. A usage protocol for the equipment may also need to be devised.
- Following qualification, a vet may decide to offer a new service to clients, which will require new protocols and procedures to be put in place.
- Newly promoted staff may need additional training to enable them to fulfil the requirements of the post.
- New legislation may require procedures to be put in place and additional monitoring to ensure compliance.
- Poor performance in the job will require the provision of additional training to enable the employee to perform better.
- Strategic plans made by management could result in training gaps arising, which need to be filled if these plans are to be achieved.

Some training can be provided on an ad hoc basis, such as a simple demonstration of how to use a new piece of equipment or how to apply new cleaning protocols, and the practice manager can usefully delegate the organization of this to supervisors or line managers. However, training that is likely to affect staffing levels or clinical rotas, or which is likely to involve a financial outlay, requires a different approach. Training needs reviews should be carried out regularly – at least once every 6 months if the practice is relatively stable, but more often in times of change. When carrying out a training needs review, practice managers should remain aware of the need for fairness and objectivity. Part-time staff have the same rights as full-time employees and should be given the same training and development opportunities, as far as is practically possible. All training needs should be assessed in relation to the wider business strategy to make sure that any training that is provided and funded contributes to the achievement of practice objectives.

A training needs review would include the following stages:

**1.** Identify the training required.

Gleaned from:

- any changes or new initiatives being planned
- results of staff appraisal meetings
- individual requests received direct.

**2.** Assess the costs versus the benefits.

- Decide how each training need might best be met and establish the associated cost (assume at this point that all training needs will be met). Even if there is in-house provision, there will still be costs associated with the training in terms of staff time or loss of practice income while staff are undergoing that training.
- Assess the benefits – these will be both tangible (e.g. increased product sales, new revenue stream, etc.) and intangible (e.g. improved staff motivation, increased efficiency, etc.).
- Decide what the practice can afford to fund, what it should fund (i.e. what is urgent) and what it cannot fund at this time. In the UK, the Royal College of Veterinary Surgeons (RCVS) requires that veterinarians undertake 35 hours of continuing professional development (CPD) each year and Registered Veterinary Nurses are required to undertake 45 hours of CPD over a 3 year period, averaging 15 hours a year (RCVS, 2011). Any staff training plan must ensure, therefore, that these obligations can be met.

**3.** Produce a prioritized list and present this to staff together with clear justification.

- It is important for staff to have the opportunity to discuss the decisions made and the reasons behind these.
- Honesty and openness are essential and will reduce feelings of disappointment or resentment considerably, especially if it is made clear that

decisions are not based on favouritism, but on sound business principles.

- Everyone must understand that training is ongoing, and while they may not have been given the go-ahead for their particular course on this occasion, it will be their turn next time.

## Meeting training needs

Training needs can be met in a variety of different ways and the method selected will be dependent on the training budget and the potential impact on the practice. The practice manager will be concerned primarily with achieving cost-effectiveness, while at the same time causing minimal disruption to the functioning of the practice and its service provision.

Private or 'home' study is by far the cheapest option for employers (Davies, 2000). Veterinarians are permitted up to 10 hours private study time as part of their 35 hours annual CPD quota. It may be possible for the staff meeting room to double up as a study room if there is sufficient space. Most staff should be able to find an hour here and there for private study, but in the interests of fairness and to ensure that all staff are treated equally, it should be possible to build private study time into the practice rotas.

E-learning or computer-aided learning is another cost-effective way to study, but one which is best suited to topics that do not require 'hands-on' experience or the demonstration of specific manual skills. For this to be successful, though, staff should be allocated the time to work through the associated DVDs or online material and should be required to demonstrate that they have completed their training, possibly through taking and passing a multiple choice question (MCQ) test or giving presentations on selected topics.

External courses should be carefully screened for price, duration, quality of content, the reputation of the organization delivering the training and the relevance of the course material. Also, an assessment should be made of how the training that is obtained will be subsequently used.

Congresses are valuable to all professionals in that they provide networking opportunities, exposure to the latest developments, clinical techniques, new equipment and products and ideas, but they are expensive in terms of time away from the practice, and travel and accommodation costs, not to mention actual congress fees. It may be possible to save on these costs through negotiating with individuals to attend part of the congress rather than the entire event, to alternate attendance year on year and to ask individuals to contribute personally to the social events, which are optional.

## Evaluating training

Whenever any training has been completed, the results should be evaluated. There are various ways of doing this:

- By asking the staff member to make a presentation to the rest of the practice team.
- By holding an informal meeting with the staff member to ask how the training went and how useful the trainee felt it was.
- If new skills were learnt, observing the staff member using these new skills.
- Testing through MCQs or practical tests.
- Asking the staff member to complete a feedback form.
- Discussing training at the staff appraisal meeting.
- Collecting feedback from colleagues and clients.

The method or methods selected will obviously depend on the type of training received and the trainee. Again, it is important to explain to staff why such monitoring is necessary and that it is not intended just to check up on them, but to assess the effectiveness of training so that better decisions and choices can be made in the future to benefit everyone. The results of such monitoring should be communicated to all staff so that those who may be reluctant to undergo training or who may not see its purpose can understand its importance and the benefits that it can bring. The results of the monitoring process, alongside other training records, can also inform budget setting for training at the start of each new financial year.

## Staff development

As has already been pointed out, staff development goes beyond training (although training usually forms a key part of development) and is about helping individuals to fulfil their true professional potential and, ideally, achieve career progression. Forsyth (2001) argues that it is a fundamental human trait to want to develop and progress, both professionally and personally, and organizations should be prepared to support this drive as long as individual and organizational objectives coincide.

Organizations can adopt varying approaches to staff development. At one end of the spectrum there is the learning organization, which actively strives to foster a 'development culture' utilizing a whole range of communication methods, which emphasize training and development activities, and involve planning and initiating new activities, reporting on their results and even including details in their annual reports (Forsyth, 2001). Such organizations have a clear structure for promotion and progression supported by annual promotion and progression reviews. At the other end of the spectrum, there is the small business, with limited resources, which is only able to provide the minimum of support, perhaps in the form of reading material or access to externally provided online resources.

Veterinary practices are often unable to offer development opportunities beyond training, although in the UK greater opportunities appear to be available if a practice is a member of the RCVS Practice Standards Scheme (PSS). Veterinary hospitals that are accredited under this Scheme are now required to have a 1 year CPD plan for the hospital team. This requirement only currently applies to veterinary hospitals though, and is not a core requirement for all veterinary practices that come under the Scheme. However, *all* PSS practices are required to have in place an annual performance review system for clinical staff in order to monitor and review their development (RCVS, 2011). Unfortunately, at this point in time, the PSS is still only voluntary.

In reality, substantial resources are not needed to foster a 'development culture' in veterinary practice, albeit on a much smaller scale, because this is really about adopting the right attitudes and behaviours. As development concerns the longer term progression of the individual, it makes sense for ownership of the process to be shared equally between the practice and its employees. Getting staff to understand their own responsibilities in this regard forms the starting point for building a 'development culture'. For such a culture to subsequently grow, however, it is essential that practice owners and managers share a fundamental belief in the value of their staff, viewing the staff as an asset that deserves investment. Practice owners and managers must:

- Share a genuine belief that staff are an asset and not an expense.

- Lead by example and be lifelong learners themselves.
- Foster good communication and information sharing throughout the practice.
- Encourage and enable staff to take responsibility for their own development.
- Put in place an effective performance appraisal system, which everyone believes in.
- Produce a written staff development policy, a copy of which is included in the staff handbook.
- Monitor and evaluate staff training and development regularly.

Following from an agreed overall approach to staff development, the written staff development policy document would include the following:

- A statement affirming the practice's commitment to staff development.
- An explanation of how this commitment will be met – the staff training plan would form a part of this.
- How staff development will be monitored and evaluated – training effectiveness monitoring would form a part of this.
- Opportunities for career progression and promotion that are available within the practice – if any.
- How often the policy will be reviewed and by whom.

In conclusion, investment in staff training and development will benefit both employees and the practice, and is an essential part of effective human resource management. A sound policy for staff development will form part of the practice's overall business strategy and will be clearly explained to staff. Training needs reviews should be carried out regularly and training should be prioritized in order to ensure that employees' needs are addressed within the overall staff development plan. Training methods should be selected both for their cost-effectiveness and potential impact on practice operations. Where there is conflict between practice and individual needs, it is important for both parties to work together to reach a suitable compromise. If this is not possible, individuals should be supported in obtaining suitable alternative employment.

## References

Business Link (2011) Why Train Your People? Available at: http://www.businesslink.gov.uk/bdotg/action/detail?itemId=1097350857&r.l1=1073858787&r.l2=1074202347&r.l3=1097344250&r.s=sc&type=RESOURCES (accessed 1 June 2012).

Cole, G.A. (2004) *Management Theory and Practice*, 6th edn. Thomson Learning, London.

Davies, C. (2000) Cost-effective CPD for part-time vets – is it possible? *In Practice* 22, 40–42

Forsyth, P. (2001) *Developing Your Staff*. Kogan Page, London.

RCVS (2011) *Practice Standards Scheme Manual*. Royal College of Veterinary Surgeons, London. Available at http://www.rcvs.org.uk/document-library/practice-standards-manual/ (accessed 4 July 2011).

Shilcock, M. (2011) How to integrate new staff members into your practice. *Veterinary Management for Today*, June 2011, 27–29.

## Revision Questions

1. Consider the needs of a newly qualified veterinary assistant and devise a suitable induction programme for them covering their first week of employment in the veterinary practice.

2. What is the purpose of an 'Induction Checklist'?

3. Explain the distinction between '*training*' and '*development*' and explain why these terms are often used interchangeably.

4. Reread the section about training needs reviews and find out whether a similar process is undertaken at your practice. If not, how does your practice manage staff training needs?

5. (a) List the 'training' activities you have recently undertaken. (b) Identify and list the 'development' activities you have recently undertaken. Draw conclusions about the predominance of one over the other and the reasons for this.

# 8 Performance Appraisal

Every employee needs to know how they are performing in their job and managers should be able to tell them using the most appropriate method, time and place. This requires an organizational culture that views regular performance feedback as a two-way process, and trained managers who are committed to the process, possess excellent interpersonal skills and are well acquainted with their employees and their employees' jobs. Langdon and Osborne (2001) argue that regular, informal feedback about performance, whether positive or negative, enables problems to be resolved straight away rather than being stored up, improves staff morale and gives employees a clear indication of where they stand. These authors argue that the formal performance appraisal, which may take place once a year, should be a culmination of this continuous feedback and, as such, would then hold no surprises for the appraisee. Johnson and Andrews (2007), reporting on research carried out at the University of Liverpool in the UK on the support needs of new veterinary graduates, found that informal reviews rather than a formal system of appraisal were more effective in preventing and reducing problems. So, if informal feedback is more effective, is there a need for formal appraisal at all? Certainly there is, because informal feedback has a number of drawbacks:

- It is unstructured.
- It is frequently undocumented.
- It is ad hoc and inconsistent.
- Not all managers are good at providing informal feedback.
- It may be forgotten.
- Informal feedback will not always relate to individual target attainment.
- It is immediate and short term.
- It tends to praise or criticize only one small aspect of performance or one task.

A formal appraisal system provides a structured and documented framework for a comprehensive review of an individual's performance over a specific review period (usually a year), and enables the identification of training needs and resources necessary for the effective future performance of a role; it is, therefore, more thorough, meaningful and lasting – at least in theory! In practice, appraisal is very difficult to implement well, primarily because it can be approached in a variety of ways and with a variety of purposes.

## What Is Performance Appraisal?

Moon (1993), cited by Wilson and Western (2000), defines appraisal as '*a formal documented system for the periodic review of an individual's performance*'. As such, appraisal is a key part of an organization's wider performance management system and is crucial to developing a shared understanding between employer and employee of what is to be achieved and how it is to be achieved to fulfil the organization's objectives (Wilson and Western, 2000). An effective performance management system will ensure that an individual's goals are closely aligned with those of the organization. Thus, the practice's objectives would be translated into team or department objectives, which, in turn, would be translated into individual objectives and targets (Fig. 8.1). In this system, performance appraisal is a means of checking the alignment of goals and of setting new individual objectives and specific targets which ensure that this alignment continues to be maintained.

Chadwick (2008) defines a successful appraisal as 'a two-way discussion that is motivational, focused, encourages improved performance and benefits the appraisee, the appraiser and the practice'. So the emphasis shifts from the alignment of objectives to motivation and encouragement, which is also the approach advocated by Shilcock and Stutchfield (2008). The individual is the focus of

© C.R. Coates 2012. *Veterinary Practice Management* (C.R. Coates)

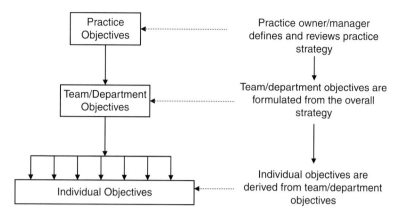

**Fig. 8.1.** Alignment of individual and practice objectives.

the formal appraisal, which is very much a dialogue with the purpose of motivating and encouraging the employee to perform better.

Many practices link performance appraisal with pay awards and/or promotion and use a scoring system for measuring individual performance. For these practices, performance appraisal is a tool for assessing the percentage pay rise an individual has earned based on past performance. Shilcock and Stutchfield (2008) argue very forcefully that appraisals should never be linked to pay as in such a system the focus of the appraisees shifts to trying to impress the boss, and they will feel inhibited and unable to be open about their jobs, which can only be detrimental to both the individual and the practice in the longer term. It could be argued, however, that without the incentive of a pay rise, employees will not take appraisals seriously and that the process will fail to motivate, but, as will be seen in the next chapter, pay is not the only motivator.

Other organizations view appraisal as a means of identifying future developmental needs, and as part of an ongoing staff development process. They view the formal appraisal primarily as a means of identifying the needs of the employee and the skills and resources that they must acquire for enhanced work performance. This could be in keeping with organizational objectives and future strategies, but alignment of individual and organizational objectives is usually taken as read in such approaches.

Thus, appraisal is a performance management tool which can be used in different ways and for different purposes:

- To ensure the alignment of individual and organizational objectives.
- To identify developmental needs.
- To motivate and encourage.
- To inform a pay review.

It is possible to use appraisal for all of these purposes at the same time, but this really requires very careful and skilful process design and is very difficult to implement correctly. This is one of the reasons why staff and managers are often not entirely clear about the purpose of appraisals and why the results of appraisals fall short of expectations. Rather than trying to achieve all these different, and at times conflicting, purposes it is best to focus on one particular objective for appraisal and for everyone to be very clear about what that is.

## The Appraisal Process

Once the purpose of appraisal has been clarified and communicated to all staff, the appraisal process can begin. In small practices, this is usually managed by one person and that person also conducts all the appraisal meetings. In larger practices, team leaders appraise their own staff, but it is essential that all appraisers receive appropriate training before conducting appraisal meetings. It is also important to ensure that the practice owners are committed to the process and are themselves appraised, either by each other or by the practice manager. As the process is time-consuming, appraisals usually take place once a year and usually at the same time each year.

The process can be broken down into the following key stages and their associated actions:

1. Pre-appraisal preparation

- Information on an individual's work performance is collected.
- Appraisal questionnaires/forms are completed.
- An agenda for the appraisal meeting is drafted.
- The date, time and location for the appraisal meeting are agreed.
- All necessary paperwork is collected (e.g. job description, last year's appraisal report, last year's action/development plan, etc.).

2. The appraisal meeting

- The individual's performance over the appraisal period is reviewed.
- Agenda items are discussed.
- Problems/barriers are identified.
- Specific achievements are identified.
- Training received is reviewed and future training needs are identified.
- An action plan is agreed, prioritized and written down, or new targets are set for the forthcoming year.
- A follow-up meeting is agreed.

3. Post-appraisal follow-up

- A report of the meeting is produced by the appraiser.
- The appraisee receives the report and comments upon/corrects factual errors.
- All appraisal documentation is collated and filed.
- The appraisee begins work on the action plan/targets.
- A follow-up meeting takes place at an appropriate time.

4. Appraisal process review

- After an appropriate interval, staff feedback on the process is collected and collated.
- Recurring themes and observations are identified.
- All documentation is reviewed.
- Action points for improvements are identified and changes/improvements to the process are put in place for the next time.
- A report is produced for all staff and circulated.

**Pre-appraisal preparation**

Information about an employee's performance during the past year can be collected in a number of different ways, depending on the purpose of the appraisal. If the purpose is primarily developmental and reflective, then it is appropriate for the appraisee to carry out a self-appraisal, which is then discussed with the appraiser. This type of appraisal is quite common in non-commercial, academic environments.

If the purpose of the appraisal is to ensure alignment with organizational objectives, then a top-down approach, in which the appraisal is carried out by the immediate manager, is appropriate.

If the purpose is performance measurement for pay awards, then information should be collected from a number of different sources. In veterinary practice, these sources could be colleagues, line managers, the practice partners or the principal. Partners can be asked to complete performance assessment forms for all staff, as well as for the other partners. Supervisors or line managers can be asked to complete forms for the staff they supervise and for other supervisors. In addition, all staff are required to complete a self-assessment form. All of the forms will include a scoring system utilizing a set of evaluative statements, for example: 1 = well above requirements; 2 = more than satisfactory; 3 = less than satisfactory; 4 = unsatisfactory. This is a time-consuming, complicated and highly subjective process, but staff may view it as being much fairer than simply being assessed by one person only and, of course, low scores driven by personal likes and dislikes will be balanced out by more objective scores.

Whichever purpose appraisal serves, both the appraiser and appraisee will need to take time to consider and to reflect upon the appraisee's performance over the review period and to collect evidence supporting this. There should be a process for collecting in the appraisal forms and collating all the necessary paperwork in plenty of time for the appraisal meeting. A period of around 2 weeks should be sufficient for the appraisee to prepare. The appraiser may have more than one appraisee and so will need more time to prepare, and because of this should be the one to suggest the date and time for the appraisal meeting.

Where a self-evaluation form is used, the appraisee can suggest topics for discussion. The form is then passed to the appraiser to read and suggest further topics. In this way, an agenda for discussion emerges.

Both parties should review the job description and any changes to the job that may have occurred over the review period. The aim is to ensure that the job description is kept up to date at all times and correctly reflects current duties and responsibilities. Also, last year's appraisal report and action plan should be revisited before the meeting.

## The appraisal meeting

This is the most important part of the appraisal process, and where the training received and personal skills of the appraiser are key. The appraiser's role is to manage the structure of the meeting, ensuring that the appraisee feels at ease and does most of the talking. The meeting will generally consist of two stages: a review of past performance, and planning future performance.

1. Review of past performance

The appraisee should be asked to report on his/her performance over the review period – identifying things that went well and things that did not go so well and the reasons for this. If the appraisee was given specific targets or had set some targets for themselves, both the appraiser and appraisee should review these together and agree an assessment of how well these had been achieved, identifying any barriers that may have prevented certain targets from being attained. It is important that the appraiser gives the appraisee a clear indication of their performance over the review period, as assessed by the appraiser and others (as applicable), and backed up by specific examples and evidence. Praise for achievements should be given. It is essential that both parties remain as objective as possible, avoid blaming others and take a constructive, forward-looking approach with the aim of improving performance and enabling the appraisee to learn from any past mistakes and failures rather than to dwell on them. It is important to identify any facilitators as well as barriers, and especially to acknowledge colleagues who have been particularly helpful or supportive.

The individual's job description should be reviewed and any significant changes to duties and responsibilities noted. If there have been significant changes, the job description should be updated following the appraisal meeting, as agreed by both parties, and including a pay review, should this be indicated.

Training and development undertaken during the review period should be noted and the effectiveness of this assessed.

2. Planning future performance

The appraisee's potential and career plans should be discussed and performance targets and measures for the forthcoming period identified and agreed. Two things are key here: (i) the appraisee should be encouraged to set his/her own targets and measures as far as practically possible, as this will ensure commitment to them; and (ii) targets should be challenging, but achievable – they need to be SMART, i.e.:

- Specific – what should be done, in what way and when.
- Measurable – in terms of the desired results.
- Achievable – fair, as agreed by both the appraiser and appraisee.
- Realistic – within the skills and capabilities of the appraisee.
- Time bound – have specific, agreed deadlines.

Once targets have been agreed, the appraiser and appraisee should draw up a plan of action together, which will enable the appraisee to comfortably achieve the agreed targets within the stipulated timescales. Any resources or additional training needed will be identified at this point. It will be up to the appraisees to take full responsibility for following the agreed plan, but to bring to their line manager's attention any issues or problems that they are unable to resolve themselves without help. If possible, a follow-up meeting should be agreed 2–3 months after the appraisal meeting to review progress.

## Post-appraisal follow-up

After the meeting, the appraiser should write a report summarizing the discussion and including details of the targets set and the action plan agreed. This should be completed as quickly as possible after the meeting and sent to the appraisee. The appraisee reads the report and requests corrections to be made, if necessary. The report is finally agreed by both parties and signed off.

The follow-up meeting with the appraisee 2 or 3 months after the appraisal meeting will review progress and discuss and resolve any problems that might have arisen since the appraisal meeting. This can be fairly informal and brief, but the appraiser must ensure that the appraisee is on track to achieve his/her targets and continues to be committed to them.

### Appraisal process review

When the appraisal process is complete, all forms and reports should be collected and filed. It is good practice to survey staff periodically to ask them how useful they felt the appraisal was. Feedback on the process from both appraisers and appraisees is crucial to ensuring its effectiveness in the future. Data should be collected from the forms and reports with the aim of identifying common issues and problems as well as good points that staff commented on most frequently. This information and the feedback collected from staff can be used as part of a review of the entire process, which should ideally be carried out by an independent person. The results of the review should be disseminated to all staff and any necessary improvements or changes should be identified and implemented straight away.

An appraisal checklist and a checklist for the appraisal meeting can be found in Section 6.

## Overcoming Staff Resistance to Appraisal

The complexity of the differing aims of appraisal and of the process itself makes it very difficult to get it right. When first introducing an appraisal system, there will inevitably be staff resistance. Reasons for this are many and varied:

- Staff may have been subjected to poorly managed appraisal in the past.
- They do not believe that a system linked to pay can be fair.
- They are suspicious of management's motives, especially if managers are not generally open with their staff.
- Promises made in the past by managers were not kept.
- Anticipated changes for the better did not happen.
- Staff do not see a need for appraisal nor understand its benefits.
- Managers view appraisal simply as a form-filling exercise.

Shilcock and Stutchfield (2008) argue that an effective appraisal system should adhere to the following principles:

- Practice owners/partners should be fully committed to the process.
- All staff should be consulted about the most appropriate format for the process.
- Appraisers should undergo appropriate training.

- The appraisal system should be kept as simple as possible.
- The system should be regularly monitored.

The main cause of performance appraisal failing is the lack of commitment to and belief in appraisal by managers, so it is essential to get the practice principal and partners on board at the outset. The best starting point is to educate people about appraisal, what it involves and what the benefits are. It is vital to decide what the primary purpose of appraisal is going to be, and this should be agreed by the majority. This process of education may take some time while arguments and counter-arguments are put forward. So long as dialogue is maintained and managers are open and honest, staff will listen. Formal training of appraisers can take place at this time and all staff should have input into deciding the type of forms to be used and the structure, timing and duration of the process. It may be necessary to bring in an external consultant to assist with setting up the system, if expertise is not available within the practice.

## References

Chadwick, A. (2008) Staff appraisals and how to do them with confidence. *The Veterinary Business Journal* No. 83, 18–20.

Johnson, B. and Andrews, F. (2007) PDP: from pilot to practice. *In Practice* 29, 166–169.

Langdon, K and Osborne, C. (2001) *Appraising Staff*, 1st edn. Dorling Kindersley, Hampton, UK.

Moon, P, (1993) *Appraising Your Staff*. Kogan Page, London.

Shilcock, M. and Stutchfield, G. (2008) *Veterinary Practice Management: A Practical Guide*, 2nd edn. Elsevier Saunders, Edinburgh, UK.

Wilson, J.P. and Western, S. (2000) Performance appraisal: an obstacle to training and development? *Career Development International* 6, 93–99.

## Revision Questions

1. Discuss the importance of appraisal as a tool for managing staff performance.

2. Develop and write down ten key rules for effective appraisals.

3. Examine the structure of an appraisal meeting and identify five key skills an appraiser should possess in order to manage the meeting effectively.

4. Discuss your views on whether appraisals should be linked to pay. Justify your viewpoint.

5. You are given the task of setting up an appraisal system for the first time. Write out an action plan detailing how you would approach this task.

# 9 Motivation

## What is Motivation?

The Oxford Dictionaries Online (2012) gives the following definition of 'motivation':

> A reason or reasons for acting or behaving in a particular way; desire or willingness to do something; enthusiasm.

If motivation is viewed as the reason why people do things, it follows that without it they would do very little indeed. Therefore, motivation is the force that drives all human action. How does motivation arise?

Hargie (2006) describes a 'needs-driven' model of human behaviour in which a person perceives that he/she has a specific need. Responding to that need, the person formulates goals (explicit or implicit) and then acts to attain them and thus to satisfy the need (Fig. 9.1).

Within this model, goals are pursued in response to their perceived importance, and motivation determines the strength with which they are pursued. At any one time, an individual will have a number of different needs, some more important than others, which they will wish to fulfil. Hargie (2006) argues that emotion plays an important mediating role in this model. It is not enough that a person knows the importance of a particular goal; that person must also have a desire or wish to pursue the goal and this emotion must be strong enough to ensure continuous action until the goal is achieved. So action is the result of a complex interplay of perceptions and needs, motivation and emotion.

Motivation is an internal state which varies both within individuals and between individuals. For example, two students undertaking the same programme of study may see themselves as pursuing the same ultimate goal (obtaining their degrees), but be motivated in entirely different ways – one might view this as the fulfilment of a lifelong dream and the other simply as a means of securing future employment.

Most people work because they need to earn money to live, but it is the type of work that they choose to do which says something about what it is that motivates them. Those with a vocational calling are motivated by their love of the work itself. For some, work is the most important thing in their lives, to the exclusion of all else – for such people work satisfies all their needs. Others simply view work as a means to an end – a way of getting the things they really want. The key for the manager in charge of staff is to try to understand what motivates each staff member as an individual and to ensure that the working environment contains sufficient motivators to build and maintain commitment.

## Theories of Workplace Motivation

Research into motivation at work has been ongoing since the 1930s and has resulted in the emergence of a number of important and influential theories, many of which are still applicable to workplaces today.

### The two-factor theory

Herzberg *et al.* (1959) identified a number of workplace factors ('satisfiers') that contribute to job satisfaction. Alongside these, a number of other factors were identified, labelled as 'hygiene factors', which have no positive effect on job satisfaction, but which increase dissatisfaction when implemented in a manner contrary to employees' expectations. The appropriate 'hygiene factors' need to be present in the workplace so as not to cause dissatisfaction, but their presence is generally taken for granted by employees (Table 9.1).

Thus, according to this theory, if employees are poorly supervised or if the working conditions are poor, they will be dissatisfied. However, if these workplace factors are good, employees will not experience any significant increase in their feelings

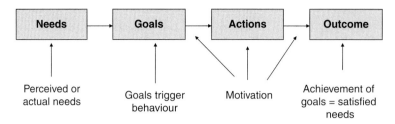

Fig. 9.1. A needs-driven model of human behaviour (adapted from Hargie, 2006).

Table 9.1. 'Satisfiers' and 'hygiene factors' – the two-factor theory (Herzberg *et al.*, 1959).

| 'Satisfiers' | 'Hygiene factors' |
| --- | --- |
| • Achievement | • Company policies |
| • Recognition | • Administration |
| • The work itself | • Supervision |
| • Responsibility | • Pay and bonuses |
| • Advancement | • Working conditions |
| | • Interpersonal relations |

of satisfaction. In contrast, satisfaction does arise from employees being given responsibility, appreciation for what they do and opportunities for growth and development.

The main criticism of this theory is that it tends to equate satisfaction with motivation, which is incorrect. Nevertheless, the 'satisfiers' clearly contribute to motivation and, thereby, are influential factors in the workplace. Managers, therefore, need to ensure that the 'satisfiers', which are within their control, are present within the working environments for which they are responsible.

### Expectancy theory

Developed by Vroom (1964), the expectancy theory makes an important link between the effort put into something, the outcome or result of that effort (referred to as 'performance') and the resulting rewards (Fig. 9.2).

The key to this model is that the person undertaking a particular effort must be clearly aware of the links and must believe that the effort they put in will be appropriately rewarded. Rewards do not have to be material or extrinsic – such as a bonus or increase in pay – to be motivating. Intrinsic rewards, such as personal satisfaction or a feeling of accomplishment, can be equally motivating. Indeed, intrinsic motivators are often more powerful than

extrinsic motivators. The key is that the individual must perceive the reward as being worth the effort. It is the person's perception of the links that creates the motivating force driving the actions. The stronger the link, the more powerful the motivating effect is. Weak links will result in poor motivation.

The factors that affect the relationship between effort, performance and rewards need to be borne in mind, however. Effort will not result in the desired outcomes if the individual lacks the ability or skills to complete the task or if he/she is unclear as to what result is expected. Also, if resources that are needed to do the job are lacking or if there is insufficient time to complete the task, motivation will be reduced because the expectation of rewards will be diminished. So it is essential that managers know their staff and their capabilities, that they are clear about their expectations and that they provide staff with the necessary resources to do their jobs.

Rewards in the form of pay increases or promotion may not be within a particular manager's power to award, but there are other ways of influencing employee motivation, such as giving recognition for work well done and providing feedback and support.

### Goal theory

Locke and Latham (1989) argue that it is the goals that individuals set for themselves that drive motivation and that specific goals are more motivating than vague or unclear goals. They discovered that there was a close correlation between setting specific and clear goals, and improvements in employee performance. In addition, they found that motivation is enhanced when feedback on performance is readily available. The concept of ownership of goals is also important here. Goals that individuals can

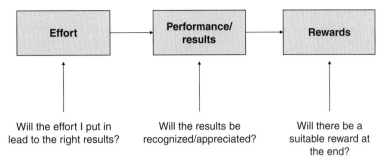

**Fig. 9.2.** The relationship between effort, results (or performance) and rewards (after Vroom, 1964).

set for themselves increase commitment and are more motivating than goals imposed by others.

### Job design – intrinsic motivation

Hackman and Oldham (1976) propose a model of job design that encompasses three key dimensions, which together determine the extent to which individuals are internally motivated to perform well in their jobs. The dimensions are skill variety, task identity and task significance; together, these determine how meaningful, worthwhile and valuable work is felt to be. The level of variety in any job has to be right, which is easier said than done. Too little variety may lead to boredom, too much variety may mean that an employee may feel unable to complete any single task well. A balance has to be struck, and this can only be achieved through careful job design and with input from the employee.

Task identity is the degree to which a job consists of complete and identifiable tasks that the employee is responsible for. The ability to complete and 'sign off' tasks in the time given helps employees to build a sense of achievement and progression. Not being able to see where one's work fits into the whole and what the results are can be demotivating. Within this model, employee autonomy is to be encouraged, as it builds a sense of ownership and responsibility for outcomes.

Task significance is the degree to which the job has a perceived value to the organization and to society as a whole. Motivation is increased if an individual perceives that his/her job is important, that it contributes to organizational objectives in a significant way and that it is worthwhile.

Conceivably, it is possible to ensure that all three dimensions are present in every job, no matter how simple. The achievement of this is really down to the experience and skill of employers and the extent to which they care about their employees.

### Pay as a Motivator

Herzberg *et al.* (1959) list pay and bonuses as one of their 'hygiene factors', arguing that a good level of pay has limited motivational potential while poor pay definitely contributes to dissatisfaction. There is evidence that the promise of a pay increase does motivate staff to better performance in the short term, but that once the increase has been awarded, the motivational effects do not last. Similarly, the real prospect of earning a bonus will inspire staff to work harder and better, but once achieved, the level of extra effort expended tends to fall.

Many employers link pay to performance and use their appraisal systems as a means of assessing the extent to which staff should be rewarded based on past performance. Depending on their performance scores, as assessed subjectively by supervisors and others, a decision is made to award a pay increase or not. This process, if perceived to be unfair, can be potentially very damaging. Staff will naturally tend to compare themselves with others, especially those on the same grade and level of pay as themselves. Any perceived unfairness is likely to lead to reduced performance, reduced commitment to the organization and, in extreme cases, staff leaving. Thus, it is vital to ensure that performance-related pay schemes are as fair as possible and to try to minimize their inherent flaws.

### Motivators and Demotivators in Veterinary Practice

The conclusions drawn by the researchers whose work is described above about motivation at work and job satisfaction are just as relevant and applicable to the veterinary practice workplace as to other workplaces.

Gazzard and Boyle (2010) report that, in general, veterinarians both here in the UK and in the USA enjoy a high level of job satisfaction, as for most of them working as a veterinarian is a lifelong dream realized. However, their survey of UK veterinary employers and employees revealed that satisfaction levels are lower for part-time workers and veterinary assistants than they are for partners, directors or sole principals. The survey also revealed that employees tend to value extrinsic factors, such as pay, holidays and favourable rotas, more highly than their employers, who value intrinsic factors, such as control over their own caseload or opportunities for progression, more highly. The authors interpret these results as a reflection of the lower career status of veterinary assistants, as they are working to meet the more basic needs. Business owners tend to enjoy higher overall job satisfaction than employees because they can control their working environment and the extrinsic and intrinsic 'satisfiers' within it; their basic needs have already been met. The message that comes across from this research, albeit of a small sample of the veterinary population, is that veterinary practice owners must pay attention to the needs of different groups of staff, so that they can work together to design a better workplace. Job satisfaction is a motivator and the presence of a good number of 'satisfiers' in the workplace acts as a powerful facilitator for managers looking to build motivation and improved work performance.

Chadwick (2008) discusses the role of the practice team leader in building motivation and recommends that leaders take the time to find out what motivates their staff, the starting point for which could be to produce a list of the top ten motivators and ask individuals to rank the list in order of importance. The information gathered in this way will only be of use, however, if staff are open and honest about what it is that motivates them.

Shouksmith and Hesketh (1986) surveyed 700 members of the New Zealand Veterinary Association to establish the levels of job and life satisfaction that they enjoyed. The results of the survey revealed that jobs were found to be particularly satisfying if they:

- were varied,
- allowed discretion,

- utilized veterinarians' skills and abilities fully,
- involved mental effort and
- allowed veterinarians to control the speed at which they worked.

When working conditions were difficult, the veterinarians tended to compensate for this by finding satisfaction in activities outside of work.

Shilcock (1999) identifies a range of motivators and demotivators present in veterinary practices. In addition to the factors identified by Herzberg *et al.* (1959) in relation to work satisfaction, communication, teamwork, a sense of belonging, listening and fair discipline act as additional motivators while poor leadership, poor communication, broken promises and working in isolation are demotivators. Shilcock (1999) also points out that if managers lack motivation themselves, then they are unlikely to be able to motivate their staff. Good communication is vital – keeping staff informed about developments and plans and asking for their input into these plans helps staff feel valued and important.

### Ensuring a Motivated Practice Team

From the foregoing, it is evident that practice owners and managers carry significant responsibility for ensuring that the veterinary practice workplace helps to build motivation and commitment, which, in turn, lead to improved performance and better outcomes both for the practice and for its staff.

To this end, managers should:

- Be motivated, enthusiastic and committed themselves.
- Respect others.
- Value their staff.
- Keep their promises.
- Know their staff – their skills, abilities and what motivates them.
- Work with staff to set clear and specific goals.
- Be clear about staff expectations.
- Provide the necessary training and resources to enable staff to do their jobs well.
- Pay fair salaries, bonuses and rewards.
- Give recognition for work well done.
- Ask for views, ideas and suggestions, and listen well.
- Provide regular, constructive feedback on performance.
- Foster good communication and good interpersonal working relationships.

- Assign responsibility and authority to staff members where appropriate.

However, managers can only really control the extrinsic motivators, as motivation is personal to the individual. Clearly, it will not be possible to motivate all staff in the same way and to the same extent, and levels of motivation will fluctuate at any one time. From time to time events outside a manager's control can occur, which will have a negative effect on motivation and job satisfaction. What is important is that managers care about their staff, their well-being and whether they are happy in their jobs, and that their staff know that they care.

## References

Chadwick, A. (2008) Cast some motivational magic on your practice. *The Veterinary Business Journal* No. 82, 20–21.

Gazzard, J. and Boyle, C. (2010) In search of better job satisfaction. *In Practice* 32, 118–121.

Hackman, J.R. and Oldham, G.R. (1976) Motivation through the design of work: test of a theory. *Organizational Behaviour and Human Performance* 16, 250–279.

Hargie, O. (2006) Skill in practice: an operational model of communicative performance. In: Hargie, O. (ed.) *The Handbook of Communication Skills*, 3rd edn. Routledge, London and New York, pp. 37–70.

Herzberg, F., Mausner, B. and Block-Snyderman, B. (1959) *The Motivation to Work*, 1st edn. John Wiley, New York.

Locke, E.A. and Latham, G.P. (1989) *A Theory of Goal-Setting and Task Performance*. Prentice-Hall, Englewood Cliffs, New Jersey.

Oxford Dictionaries Online (2012) Available at: http://oxforddictionaries.com/definition/motivation?q=motivation (accessed 1 June 2012).

Shilcock, M. (1999) Motivation – why and how? *In Practice* 21, 397–401.

Shouksmith, G. and Hesketh, B. (1986) Changing horses in mid-stream: job and life satisfaction for veterinarians. *New Zealand Veterinary Journal* 34, 141–144.

Vroom, V. (1964) *Work and Motivation*. John Wiley, New York.

## Revision Questions

**1.** Applying Herzberg's two-factor theory, identify three 'satisfiers' and three 'hygiene factors' relevant to your own present situation.

**2.** Consider a time when you worked particularly hard to achieve a goal. Identify what it was that motivated you to put in this effort and distinguish between extrinsic and intrinsic motivators.

**3.** Based on Hackman and Oldham's (1976) 'job design' theory, describe what would be your ideal job in veterinary practice.

**4.** Identify three ways in which managers can influence intrinsic motivation.

# 10 Leadership and Management – Do You Have What it Takes?

In today's world everyone experiences leadership every day at various levels and in a variety of ways. Here are some examples:

- Citizens are directly and indirectly affected by the decisions made by their country's leaders whom they elected to represent them.
- Employees are directly and indirectly affected by the decisions made by organizational heads, business owners, directors and managers who hold positions of authority over them.
- In sport, team captains lead, team members follow.
- In education, students are led by programme directors, subject managers, teachers and administrators.
- Members of recreational clubs and societies elect individuals to lead them and make decisions on their behalf.

The practice of leadership is universal and ubiquitous. Often it is done well, but equally often it is done badly. Researchers have tried for a long time to find out what it is that makes an effective leader and whether this can be taught and learnt. Indeed, leadership has been studied extensively within a variety of different contexts, cultures and theoretical frameworks, resulting in a considerable body of knowledge (Horner, 1997). The modern view, however, is succinctly summarized by Conger (2004), who states that good leaders are born *and* made. In other words, it is the combination of an individual's genetic predisposition, life experiences (including family environment, school, hardships, jobs) and training that determine the type of leader that a person will become, assuming that they want to lead. Conger identifies high energy levels and above average cognitive abilities as being critical to effective leadership. He also argues that later experiences will continue to influence and shape a person's talents and abilities, particularly hardship or intense challenges that are faced. Thus,

experience also plays an important role in the development of leadership skills.

Leaders do not operate in isolation or in a vacuum. They need followers to follow them and environments within which to exercise their talents and make decisions. The effectiveness of leadership, therefore, is a complex interplay of the individual leader, his/her followers and the context within which the leader–follower relationship proceeds. Therefore, a range of factors has an influence on the effectiveness of leadership. In a world of rapid change where organizations are no longer stable or static, today's working environments are complex and continually evolving. Leaders now have to deal with greater challenges than ever before, which requires them to be versatile and adaptable and to have the ability to vary their leadership style to fit the changing circumstances.

## The Distinction Between Management and Leadership

The functions of leadership and management are often viewed as synonymous, largely because managers are often leaders and vice versa. But, strictly speaking, these two roles are not the same and it is important to be clear about this. Leadership generally concerns itself with the bigger picture, i.e. defining future strategies and objectives and maintaining a holistic view of the organization or business. Leadership provides a vision and creates and builds the culture of the organization. Leaders motivate and inspire and are responsible for generating organizational policies and rules (Fig. 10.1).

Management's role is to translate leadership vision, plans and ideas into workable departmental, team and individual objectives. Managers are responsible for developing and implementing protocols and overseeing their implementation. They direct and control staff, monitor workflows and productivity and make operational decisions.

© C.R. Coates 2012. *Veterinary Practice Management* (C.R. Coates)

So while leaders are concerned with the bigger picture, the managers' role is to ensure that their vision is implemented in the most effective way. Managers also act as an important link between leaders and staff (Fig. 10.2).

In veterinary practice, the owners provide the vision and leadership, but often also manage the practice, so they perform both roles. Not all practices have a practice manager, which may be counterproductive, because a good practice manager will allow the owners to focus on leadership while others take care of the day-to-day functioning of the practice. However, a practice manager may also be expected to perform several leadership functions, depending on the amount of responsibility and authority that the owners delegate to them and on the owners' understanding and perception of the leadership role. Thus, in veterinary practice, the distinction between leadership and management is often blurred. What is important for a successful practice, though, is that owners and managers are fully aware of their leadership role and do not neglect it. What often happens is that both owners and managers know how to manage, but not how to lead their teams effectively.

## Leadership Characteristics and Skills

Little (2011) does not make a distinction between leadership and management when listing the leadership traits which are, in his view, the most important for leading veterinary teams:

- **Vision** – Knowing where one wants to go and sharing this vision with the team. Explaining future plans and the reasoning behind these. Having clear objectives and celebrating their successful attainment along the way.
- **Toughness** – Not being afraid to deal with conflict, make difficult decisions or discipline staff.

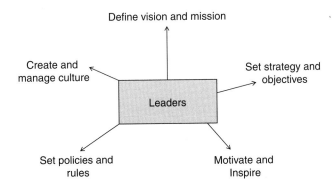

**Fig. 10.1.** What leaders do.

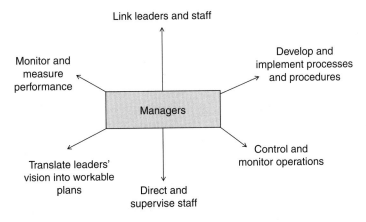

**Fig. 10.2.** What managers do.

Having the ability to cope when times are hard and to change tack, if necessary.

- **Integrity and warmth** – Caring about people, honesty, being fair in all dealings with others, able to maintain confidentiality when appropriate, always acting from the best motives, keeping promises made.
- **Enthusiasm** – Pursuing goals with vigour and energy, caring about everything one does, having faith in one's vision.
- **Knowing the team** – Knowing the strengths of each team member and utilizing their skills and aptitudes fully.
- **Building and leading the team** – Appreciating everyone's contribution and ensuring that everyone is heard. Allowing autonomy in decision making and responsibility when appropriate. Giving the team the resources, confidence and freedom to make decisions and function effectively in one's absence.
- **Motivating the team** – Instilling enthusiasm and a sense of purpose, providing appropriate motivators for team members.
- **Enhancing commitment** – Communicating well, creating a sense of belonging, showing appreciation and giving positive feedback.
- **Delegating effectively** – Identifying the right people to delegate to and then giving them the responsibility, authority and resources to carry out delegated tasks. The ability to recognize when support is needed by delegatees and when they can be left alone to get on with the job.

For Little (2011) effective veterinary team leadership, therefore, involves a combination of key internal traits, such as integrity, warmth, enthusiasm and an interest in others, and external team-building skills, such as the ability to motivate, enthuse and delegate. Little points out that it is unlikely that one individual will possess all of these traits, but that the leadership function can be shared, so that the strengths of one partner, for example, could be complemented by the different strengths of another, if the practice has more than one partner.

Coffman (2002) stresses the importance of interpersonal skills to the success of private practice, because service is the essence of a veterinarian's work. Hence, the ability to communicate effectively and to build and maintain personal and professional relationships with people from diverse backgrounds and cultures is a crucial leadership

skill. Burge (2003) supports this view, pointing out that veterinarians must lead and manage not only hospital staff, but also pet owners; and that to apply their expertise to achieve the best possible outcomes, they need to be highly skilled in the art of getting things done through others.

Burge (2003) cites the research of Goleman (1995, 1998), which demonstrates a clear link between successful leadership and high levels of emotional intelligence. Emotional intelligence (EI) refers to a person's ability to manage their own emotions and to accurately recognize the emotions of others. Managers who score highly in EI tests have high levels of self-awareness, are able to understand and manage their own emotions and to use that understanding to deal with situations in a productive and positive way. Such individuals are also self-motivated and possess an ability to thrive on adversity as well as to benefit from opportunity. They relate well to others and are effective communicators (Myers and Tucker, 2005).

Humble (2001) cites Kouzes and Posner (1987) who identify five practices that successful leaders have in common:

1. Challenging the process
2. Inspiring a shared vision
3. Enabling others to act
4. Modelling the way
5. Encouraging the heart.

Although Humble does not elaborate on these five practices, they refer to how a leader should behave, thus shifting the focus from internal traits to behaviours. Inspiring others to share the same vision, and enabling and encouraging one's team have already been mentioned. Add to these leading by example and challenging the status quo with the aim of improving team effectiveness, which are additional behaviours exhibited by effective leaders.

In the UK, the Council for Excellence in Management and Leadership (CEML) set up an SME (small and medium-sized businesses) working party, which commissioned research aimed at finding out how entrepreneurs (i.e. business owners) and their staff develop management and leadership abilities. The results of this research were published in a report in 2002 (Perren and Grant, 2002). A small group of entrepreneurs and managers from diverse industries were asked what they thought were the key management and leadership abilities that are needed in SMEs. The following were identified most frequently by the entrepreneurs:

- Ability to inspire, motivate and engender action
- Communication
- Leading by example, from the front
- Passion, drive and energy
- Clear vision, strategy, goal setting
- Ability to learn as you go
- Questioning
- Humility, open mindedness, sensitivity and self-understanding.

The managers also identified motivation, communication and team building as key skills, but for them, technical abilities and knowledge, such as organizing, training and development, knowledge of the industry, technical knowledge, accounting and budgetary control, were deemed to be more important, indicating that in SMEs, at least, there still is a strong distinction between the functions of leadership and management. Unfortunately, no attempt was made either in the questions asked or in the responses given to separate out the management skills from the leadership skills, which is a shortcoming of this research.

Clearly, there is no one definitive set of leadership skills and abilities that could be claimed to apply to all leaders, irrespective of position, industry or organizational context, the primary reason for this being the role that context plays in determining the types of abilities and skills that are most useful. Therefore, in different settings and environments, different abilities and skills are needed. An effective leader is one who can adapt to the environment and bring to bear the most appropriate skills. However, two particular skills that can be said to be universal are interpersonal and communication skills, and all managers need to work to develop a high level of both.

### How Can Managers Acquire and Develop Leadership Skills?

The CEML study also asked entrepreneurs and managers how they developed their management and leadership abilities and what leadership and management development should be provided that would be most useful to them. Entrepreneurs developed their skills by informal means, such as observing management practices in other firms and informal mentoring by a more experienced person. There were also many development opportunities within their day-to-day work and arising from contacts with other entrepreneurs and managers.

Interestingly, the entrepreneurs perceived these informal means to be more useful than formal management courses, which some of them had attended. Most of the managers, in contrast, had received some form of formal training, ranging from a 2 day course through to a master's degree, indicating that for the managers this type of learning was seen as important. However, they also put a high value on informal mentorship and observing the practices of others.

As to what leadership and management development should be provided, the entrepreneurs listed informal mentoring and learning from peers and business coaching as their most preferred forms of development. While they did not rule out formal courses and training, they asked for courses tailored to their specific needs which could be completed in a flexible way, because lack of time was an issue. The managers expressed a preference for formal, short courses, but wanted these to be available at more convenient times and on specific topics, such as health and safety management, assertiveness, retailing, accounting and marketing.

Thus, it appears that, for these entrepreneurs and managers at least, formal courses are not as effective or as valued as informal means of learning. High on the list of effective informal methods are mentoring and peer support, and so leaders and managers should actively build links with other leaders and managers and seek out suitable mentors. One obvious way to do this is to join and actively participate in professional associations, congresses and e-groups, which enable daily contact with other like-minded individuals as well as providing networking opportunities.

Formal training courses do have a role to play, but these should be selected carefully specifically for their relevance to a manager's current situation, flexibility of delivery and the certainty that what is learnt will be immediately utilized at work.

The crucial role of varied personal and professional experience for effective leadership has already been mentioned. It follows that managers who wish to excel as leaders should actively seek different and greater challenges and grasp opportunities as they arise. An area where experience is particularly useful and pertinent is people management. Out-of-work activities, such as membership of sports teams, clubs and societies, and opportunities for public speaking, will also contribute to the development of interpersonal and communication skills.

Coffman (2002) argues that the problem-solving skills that veterinarians utilize in day-to-day practice can also be applied elsewhere – for example, in dispute resolution and when dealing with employee complaints or grievances. This methodical diagnostic process, according to Coffman (2002), can form the basis of fair decision making in any situation. So veterinarians have a strong advantage over other managers, in that they arrive already equipped with an effective decision-making tool which they are practised at using. The veterinarian's consummate professionalism also serves them well in leadership roles.

Veterinary and veterinary nursing students have the opportunity to gain and develop key management and leadership skills while at university:

- Through membership and leadership of small groups and teams throughout their time at university
- Membership and leadership of sports teams and student societies
- Membership and leadership of the students' union
- Preparing and giving presentations
- Organizing and carrying out projects
- Representing their fellow students as year representatives
- Representing their fellow students in staff–student liaison meetings
- Meeting and dealing with clients during their clinical years
- As part of formal units of study, which include leadership and management training.

University is a safe environment in which to acquire and practise these skills before going out into the world of work. Those who lack such valuable experience – either out of choice or a lack of opportunity – should seek ways to correct this situation, because a student who has gained a range of different experiences and skills will be a more attractive candidate for potential employers.

Innate traits, such as enthusiasm, passion, drive and integrity, cannot really be taught – they are either present or not. Their absence may have as much to do with the environment and the position held as with the individual manager's own disposition and character. It is up to the manager to decide which is the prevailing influence and, if necessary, to change jobs, seeking out a position and environment that suits their personality better.

## References

Burge, G.D. (2003) Six barriers to veterinary career success. *Journal of Veterinary Medical Education* 30, 1–4.

Coffman, J. R. (2002) Veterinary medical education and a changing culture. *Journal of Veterinary Medical Education* 29, 66–70.

Conger, J.A. (2004) Developing leadership capability: what's inside the black box? *The Academy of Management Executive (1993–2005)* 18, 136–139.

Goleman D. (1995) *Emotional Intelligence*. Bantam, New York.

Goleman D. (1998) *Working with Emotional Intelligence*. Bantam, New York.

Horner, M. (1997) Leadership theory: past, present and future. *Team Performance Management* 3, 270–287.

Humble, J.A. (2001) Critical skills for future veterinarians. *Journal of Veterinary Medical Education* 28, 50–53.

Kouzes, J.M. and Posner, B.Z. (1987) *The Leadership Challenge*. Jossey-Bass, San Francisco, California.

Little, G. (2011) Taking the lead: heading a team successfully. *In Practice* 33, 138–140.

Myers, L.L. and Tucker, M.L. (2005) Increasing awareness of emotional intelligence in a business curriculum. *Business Communication Quarterly* 68, 44–51.

Perren, L. and Grant, P. (2002) *Management and Leadership in UK SMEs: Witness Testimonies from the World of Entrepreneurs and SME Managers*. Report by the SME Working Group, Council for Excellence in Management and Leadership, London. Available at http://www.managementandleadershipcouncil.org/downloads/r4.pdf (accessed 7 April 2012).

## Revision Questions

**1.** Reread the above chapter and draw up a table headed 'Traits and Behaviours of Effective Leaders'. Complete your table by listing as many innate traits and leadership behaviours or practices as you can.

**2.** Reflect on your own personal and professional experience and identify the specific management and leadership skills that you have acquired/continue to acquire.

**3.** Write a brief assessment (maximum 200 words) of the importance of good leadership in ensuring practice profitability.

**4.** Identify the leadership abilities that are most applicable to your current situation and the ways in which you plan to develop these over the next 6 months.

# SECTION 3
# Working Efficiently and Effectively: Internal Processes and Procedures

## Section Objectives

At the end of this section, you should be able to:

- Explain and apply a standard procedure for implementing practice protocols.
- Understand the principles of health and safety management.
- Explain how health and safety should be managed in a veterinary practice.
- Understand the importance of good stock management and explain the principles.
- Carry out an audit of current stock management procedures and recommend improvements.
- Understand and explain the role of practice computer systems.
- Manage the selection and implementation of a new practice computer system.
- Explain the measures that managers need to take to ensure system security and legality.

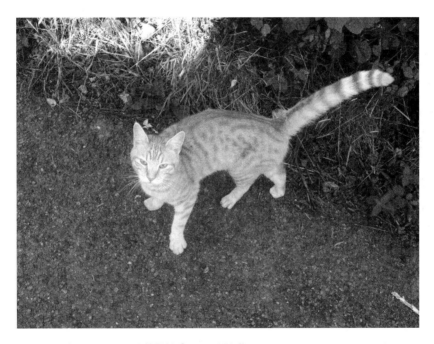

Cats are the UK's second favourite animal (PFMA Survey, 2011).

# 11 Practice Protocols and Procedures

The primary function of a veterinary practice is underpinned by a range of different protocols and procedures, which ensure its smooth functioning day to day. Effective protocols and standard operating procedures (SOPs) are essential, because without them there would be chaos and the practice would probably be a dangerous place to work at. Gunn (2000) defines SOPs as '*written documents describing routine procedures carried out*', but a more accurate definition would be '*agreed ways of doing things, which are documented and reviewed regularly*'. SOPs are needed in a veterinary practice in order to:

- Ensure compliance with legislation, e.g. health and safety regulations, veterinary medicines regulations, data protection, fire safety regulations, etc.
- Prevent duplication of effort.
- Ensure consistency in service provision.
- Help new staff settle into their jobs more quickly and smoothly.
- Help existing staff carry out their duties effectively and safely.
- Protect the practice, its staff and clients.
- Monitor and improve efficiency and effectiveness.

'Efficiency' refers to the way in which things are done. 'Effectiveness' refers to the results or outcomes. So, practices seek to carry out tasks in a timely manner that utilizes optimum levels of physical and human resources (efficiency) in order to obtain the desired results both for the practice and the pets under their care (effectiveness).

Examples of management and administrative tasks which are governed by set procedures within a veterinary practice are shown in Table 11.1. Most of these tasks and procedures are governed by legislation and are the responsibility of the practice owners. If a practice has a practice manager, the owners may delegate the tasks to that person, but would still retain overall responsibility.

Clinical procedures are the domain of the veterinarian and veterinary nurse who are trained professionals, but in order to ensure a high standard of clinical care and service provision, these staff should carry out regular clinical audits.

Health and safety procedures, stock management and information technology management are discussed in the remaining chapters of this section.

## Financial Procedures

All businesses are required to record their financial transactions in accordance with the rules of accounting, which are regulated by UK Generally Accepted Accounting Practice (GAAP) (Institute of Certified Bookkeepers, 2009). This means that an appropriate system of recording needs to be in place and that certain procedures must be followed. Accounting software is available which enables computerized record keeping and payroll management.

### Practice income

All payments made by clients are recorded on the practice computer system. The data are then transferred to the accounting system. Receptionists should ensure that all cash, cheques and credit card slips collected during the working day are kept in a safe place, which is usually a lockable till, kept hidden from client view and locked whenever the reception area is unmanned. At the end of the day, a cashing up procedure is carried out whereby the contents of the till are reconciled with a summary printout produced by the practice computer system; any discrepancies are investigated and resolved. The contents of the till are then transferred to the practice safe to await the banking procedure or they are banked on the same day. A record of cash and cheques taken to the bank is made using appropriate banking forms, which the bank countersigns and stamps. A receipt is issued for the cash and this is kept on file as evidence. The practice manager or

**Table 11.1.** Management and administrative tasks within a veterinary practice that are governed by set procedures.

| Task | Procedure |
|---|---|
| Human resource management | • Recruitment<br>• Induction training<br>• Appraisals<br>• Disciplinary and grievance<br>• Redundancy<br>• Pay and Pensions<br>• Taxation<br>• Expenses claims processing |
| Financial management | • Bookkeeping<br>• Production of monthly and year-end accounts<br>• Safeguarding practice cash<br>• Banking cash<br>• Ordering drugs and consumables<br>• Purchasing equipment<br>• Invoicing<br>• Debt control |
| General management | • Rotas<br>• Security of buildings and contents<br>• Stock control<br>• Health and safety<br>• Fire safety<br>• Radiation safety<br>• Waste disposal |
| Information technology management | • Backups<br>• System administration<br>• Generation of management data<br>• User training<br>• Data protection |

administrator will check the work of the receptionists and record the amounts banked on to the accounting system. Nowadays, veterinary practices do not collect or hold large amounts of cash as most clients prefer to pay by credit or debit card. Nevertheless, maintaining the security of cash that remains on the premises is essential and staff should be trained to handle cash correctly, to safeguard the till and to ensure that safe keys are always kept in a secure location when not in use.

### Practice expenditure

Ordering of drugs and consumables is often the designated duty of the Head Nurse. All orders placed with suppliers should be numbered and dated. Drugs orders can be placed with suppliers online, but it is essential to keep a copy of orders that have been made, either in paper or electronic form. There is a special procedure for ordering controlled drugs, which has to be supervised by a veterinarian. It is good practice to give the nurse an expenditure limit for orders, so that when that limit has to be exceeded, the order will then need to be authorized by a more senior member of staff who should carry out any necessary checks before approving the order. This imposes controls on purchasing and increases awareness of costs and spending.

When the goods are delivered, they should be unpacked immediately and carefully checked against the order and delivery note accompanying them. Any discrepancies should be notified to the supplier and a note placed on the paperwork detailing the nature of the discrepancy and how it is to be remedied. Once the delivery has been checked and the paperwork signed, the goods can be placed on the shelves or in their designated storage area. A barcode system speeds up the ordering and delivery process and enables drug stocks to be automatically updated on the computer system.

When the invoice arrives from the supplier, this should be checked against the order and delivery note by a person other than the person who placed the order. This ensures that ordering and invoice approval are not in the hands of one person, thus protecting staff as well as the practice. Details of orders placed, delivery notes and invoices paid are entered into the accounts software and payments to suppliers are made according to suppliers' credit terms by bank transfer, utilizing secure online facilities.

It is essential that practice owners carry out an audit of all financial procedures at least once a year, with the help of the accountant, if necessary. Such an audit would include, among other things, following a number of randomly selected transactions from the ordering stage through delivery to invoice payment in order to ensure that:

• all the necessary paperwork is present;
• the essential checks were correctly carried out by staff;
• any discrepancies were resolved; and
• the invoice was correct and paid at the proper time.

## Credit Control

Most small animal practices operate a 'payment at the time of treatment' policy, which is relatively easy to enforce, but large animal and equine practices are obliged to invoice their clients, usually after a veterinarian has visited a farm or yard. Inevitably, with larger numbers of invoices being issued, there is a greater likelihood of a percentage of these remaining unpaid and the practice needs to have a procedure in place for handling outstanding debts.

By far the best approach is to avoid debts occurring in the first place by ensuring that all new clients are informed about the practice's policy regarding payment. Shilcock and Stutchfield (2008) advise that written *'terms and conditions of business'* should be given to all new clients, either separately or included in the practice brochure. Dingwall (2007) recommends that this information be included as part of a 'Client Welcome Pack'. The practice's written terms and conditions of business should include:

- A clear policy statement about payment, e.g. 'It is the policy of this practice to collect payment at the time of treatment, as no credit can be given'.
- Details of any interest that the practice charges for late payments or overdue accounts.
- An outline of the procedure the practice follows to obtain payment, including the use of debt collection agencies and/or solicitors.
- Contact details for the person in charge of credit control in the practice.
- Information about organizations and charities that are able to provide financial support to clients on low incomes.

Hopps (2008) suggests that practices should carry out credit checks on new clients and ask them for references. Clients should be familiar with such a policy and should not consider it an unfair request, but it may not be possible for practices to do this as routine or, in particular, for small animal practice clients who only ever intend to bring their pets to the practice for annual health checks and vaccinations, as it may seem excessive and may well put them off registering. However, for large animal and equine practices that have many business clients (farmers, livery yard owners, etc.), such a policy is justifiable.

All invoices should be sent out to clients as soon as possible after treatment with a 'pay by' date clearly shown. Dingwall (2007) recommends invoicing more frequently for equine clients (say, weekly rather than monthly), because if a veterinarian's visit is still fresh in a client's mind, they are less likely to disagree with the practice's charges. All invoices should contain the following essential information:

- Invoice number
- Date
- VAT registration number
- Name and address of practice
- Name and address of client
- Description of the service provided and the net costs
- Name, quantity, dosage and net cost of any drugs or medicines supplied
- Total net price
- VAT rate and amount of VAT charged
- Total amount due
- Payment terms – e.g. *'Payment is required by return'*
- Methods by which payment can be made.

Copies of all invoices sent out to clients should be kept on file and retained in the practice (even when paid) for a period of at least 6 years.

Practices will vary in their preferred method of collecting debts. What is important is that the procedure is followed consistently, methodically and routinely, that it is well documented and that all staff are familiar with it. It should also enable anyone filling in for the credit controller to complete the necessary tasks in their absence. Staff awareness and training are crucial. McNeill and Blayney (2007) argue that all staff, including partners, should be required to follow the procedures without exception, with any deliberate failure to do so resulting in disciplinary action.

It is hardly worth pursuing payment of a debt that is unlikely to be paid so a first step should be to contact the client by telephone and talk to them about it to establish whether they are likely to pay, when payment will be made or if they are experiencing any difficulties with which the practice may be able to help. This task should be carried out by an experienced member of staff who is able to ask for money skilfully and tactfully.

Written client reminders for outstanding debts are used by many practices. Hughes (2010) recommends that practices send out no more than three consecutive reminders, and that they should follow each one up with a telephone call. Then, if the bill remains unpaid, the use of a debt collection agency should be considered. The debt collection agency chosen should have an excellent track record of success and a variety of investigative tools at its disposal which can enable it to gather sufficient information about the client and the client's credit history and current credit status to reach an informed decision about whether to pursue the debt or write it off.

For debts over £100 and up to a value of £5000 it may be necessary, as a last resort, to start a claim through the Small Claims Court (SSC). This involves completing a form and sending it with a fee to the local county court. The practice then becomes the 'claimant' and the debtor the 'defendant'. The court will contact the defendant, setting out the options available and the timescale involved. The defendant can make arrangements to pay at this point. If no payment is forthcoming, the claimant will then issue a Request for Judgment. In response, the court will issue a Judgment for Claimant and send it to the defendant. This represents an order to the defendant to pay. This judgment will also be entered into the public register, the effect of which is that the defendant may find it very difficult to obtain credit from anyone in the future.

Clearly, resorting to court proceedings is time-consuming and costly, not to mention the ill will that it will generate, so before starting the process, practices need to ensure that there is a high likelihood of success. Thus, clients who are pursued in this way would normally be those who clearly have the funds to pay, but do not pay because of an unjustified dispute with the practice. In such cases, the practice must be certain that the pursuit is fully justified and that it has done everything in its power to clear up any misunderstandings and answer any criticisms from the client beforehand.

## Record Keeping

During the course of its day-to-day business a practice will generate a large number of different types of records. Financial records need to be kept for a period of at least 6 years, which has implications for filing and storage, so a methodical and organized filing system needs to be in place. Older records can be stored in a locked store room, but in such a way that enables easy access to them for audit purposes. Records older than 6 years can be shredded and handed over to a recycling contractor. At the end of each financial year, the practice manager should file away the year's records and

shred and discard those that are no longer needed. This should become a routine annual procedure. This is an important responsibility, because ignoring it can result in excessive amounts of paperwork occupying space unnecessarily and becoming a fire hazard.

Retention of staff records is a complex and ever-changing area of human resource management (Chartered Institute of Personnel and Development, 2011). In the UK, the storage and retention of such records is governed by a combination of European Union (EU) and UK legislation. The Data Protection Act 1998 is the key statutory instrument; this requires every employer to have an 'appropriate filing system' in place, which is confidential, secure and to which access is limited to key personnel only. Records must be accurate, kept up to date and used only for the purposes for which they were intended. Individuals are permitted access to their own records under the provisions of the Act and are entitled to request that inaccurate information be amended.

Client records are also covered by the provisions of the Data Protection Act 1998. Accordingly, clients are allowed to view the records that a practice holds about them and their pets. Because of this right, all staff should ensure that entries made into the practice computer system about clients and their animals are factual, accurate and truthful. In addition, staff should be trained in maintaining confidentiality – not to discuss clients with people outside the practice and not to give out information to third parties without the express permission of the client. Receptionists should be provided with guidance on how to deal with a client request to view records. Clients may, from time to time, ask for copies of X-rays or other records. X-rays are the property of the practice and this must be made clear to clients, but copies can be made and given to clients on request. A reasonable charge for this service can be made to cover the costs that the practice incurs.

## Developing SOPs

When practice procedures and SOPs work well, the practice functions smoothly – staff know what to do at all times and clients view the practice as an efficient and effective operation. However, from time to time, signs may begin to appear signalling that all is not well and that a protocol or procedure is needed. Common signals include:

- When clients complain of conflicting advice or inconsistent treatment being given.
- When frequent errors are made or the same error is repeated.
- When some jobs do not seem to be anyone's responsibility.
- When vital equipment or paperwork is difficult to locate.
- When certain tasks seem to take longer than they should.

It is essential to establish what is going wrong, identify the cause and take steps to remedy the problem. If a new procedure is the remedy, certain key questions need to be addressed:

- What protocol/procedure is needed here?
- Why do we need it?
- Who will be expected to follow it?
- Does the protocol/procedure need to be written down?
- Who should write it down?
- Where will copies be kept and how will staff access them?
- Who is going to review and update the procedure?
- How often should it be reviewed?
- Should there be any penalties if staff fail to comply with it?

A template for developing a new procedure can be found in Section 6.

The person whose job it is to develop the procedure should involve relevant team members in the process in order to gain their views and ideas and to build a comprehensive picture of how the new procedure will work. A first draft should be written up and shown to the team. Team members should work through the procedure to test it. Testing will reveal whether any changes need to be made before it is finalized.

Once a new procedure is implemented and given time to bed in, staff should be asked for their views on how it is working. If all is well, a review date can be set, as appropriate. Procedures that are required to be put in place by law must be adhered to by all staff. These still need to be thought through in the way described before implementation, but non-compliance should carry a penalty, either in the form of disciplinary action or a reprimand, depending on the severity of the transgression.

In conclusion, protocols and procedures are an essential part of business life. Protocols should be developed to reflect best practice and should be aimed at improving a practice's overall efficiency and effectiveness. Physical and staffing resources should be utilized carefully. Staff should understand the purpose of and need for protocols, which should never be over-prescriptive or controlling. Finally, protocols should be enabling, not limiting. Regular reviews of standard practice procedures should help to avoid this.

## References

Chartered Institute of Personnel and Development (2011). Retention of HR Records: Resource summary. Available at: http://www.cipd.co.uk/hr-resources/factsheets/retention-hr-records.aspx (accessed 13 September 2011).

Dingwall, R. (2007) Debt: is it the hidden enemy in your practice? *The Veterinary Business Journal* No. 77, 12–14.

Gunn, D. (2000) Standard operating procedures – the why and the how. *In Practice* 22, 343–344.

Hopps, B. (2008) Advice for collecting debts in a tight market. *The Veterinary Business Journal* No. 86, 44–45.

Hughes, C. (2010) Debt collection: top tips for getting what you're owed. *The Veterinary Business Journal* No. 95, 30–31.

Institute of Certified Bookkeepers (2009) *Advanced Bookkeeping*, Kaplan, Wokingham, UK.

McNeill, E. and Blayney, N. (2007) Can't pay? Won't pay? Managing debt in practice. *In Practice* 29, 47–50.

Shilcock, M. and Stutchfield, G. (2008) *Veterinary Practice Management: A Practical Guide*, 2nd edn. Saunders Elsevier, Edinburgh, UK.

## Revision Questions

1. Select a practice procedure with which you are familiar and decide whether it works well for you. If so, identify the factors that make it work. If not, how might it be improved?

2. You have been given the task of writing a procedure for the receptionists for dealing with emergency calls. Outline the approach you would take to this task and produce a flow chart of the procedure.

3. Do all practice procedures need to be written down? Identify three procedures, which are followed in your practice, but which are not written down. Explain the reasons why they do not need to be written down.

4. Explain how you would deal with a client's request for a copy of his/her pet's records.

# 12 Principles of Health and Safety

## ALAN JONES

Workplace safety is not just a management responsibility. It involves the whole practice staff working in the safest way that they can. The legislation is specific in some areas and general in others, but because there may not be any specific legislation on some areas of the practice, all staff should work together to ensure that everyone contributes to safe working by following a duty of care to colleagues, clients and visitors.

In this chapter, I have deliberately not referenced every comment, but have included a list of useful web sites at the end. Specific detail of the legislation has been omitted because, in my opinion, learning legislation off by heart does not make for a safe working environment. What does make a safe working environment is thinking about how the environment and working practices can be improved to reduce the risks and improve patient care at the same time. Reviewing risk assessments, learning from experience and regularly updating methods of working are the best ways of continuously improving the safety of a practice.

## General Principles

Health and safety in the clinical environment is much more than following legal requirements and filling out appropriate paperwork. It involves clinical skill, consideration of the client and patient populations, and the commitment of all staff in the practice to ensuring that the environment is as safe as possible to work in by instilling good practice and extending this good practice ethos to patient care as well.

The range of issues that require consideration under the general banner of health and safety in clinical practice is an eclectic mixture, with the types of legislative knowledge, especially detailed knowledge, that are required being determined by the client and patient base of the practice. A practice that has small animal patients is not likely to have the same potential hazards as an equine or farm animal practice. For this reason, the interpretation of the legislation and implementation of safe working practices requires a good understanding of the hazards and risks associated with the particular area/s of veterinary clinical practice concerned.

For the purposes of health and safety, it is necessary to examine the ways that clinical work is carried out. This analytical process can often highlight where improvements can be made. If we consider, for example, the simple task of moving a patient from a kennel to the induction room before orthopaedic surgery, we can use the principles of health and safety to aid our planning process for the safe movement of the patient. If the patient is in pain from a fracture or nerve compression, sharp or sudden movements may increase pain and give rise to the patient defending itself in an attempt to stop the pain. The patient may yelp or bite to ensure that it is not disturbed, which could result in a member of the care team being bitten. To reduce this risk we need to consider how many people are needed and are available to move the patient and how practised the team is at working in a coordinated manner. We also need to consider whether the patient requires additional analgesia before it is moved, because even slight movements in the wrong plane can elicit excruciating pain for brief periods with, for example, nerve compression injuries. The method of transport from the kennel to the induction room is also an important consideration. Are we going to use a trolley or a stretcher? Either may cause jolting of the patient. Are there doors that need to be opened en route? If so, the journey should be planned so that there is as little change of momentum as possible. Although the focus here is primarily on the patient, by looking after the patient's needs we are reducing the risk of injury to staff, so by considering the patient we are using the same process to ensure the safety of staff.

Where patients are concerned, the same assessment process can be used to ensure that no harm is done by taking account of not only the treatments,

© C.R. Coates 2012. *Veterinary Practice Management* (C.R. Coates)

but also of simple tasks, such as manual handling and the environment. In this context, the environment may mean not only the *gross environment*, such as practice buildings, their layout and facilities, but also the *micro-environment*, such as the area immediately surrounding a patient on an operating table.

## Legal Requirements

The introduction of health and safety legislation goes back to the period of industrial reforms when mechanization started to take over from manual skills and cottage industry, with a subsequent increase in the frequency of work-related injuries. Improvements to the working environment over time led to a reduction in the severity and frequency of industrial injuries not only in high-risk jobs, but also in the caring professions. Along with the introduction of specific legislation, there is a common theme of education and cultural change within the workplace. The most significant cultural change and legislative requirement has been the formal recording of work processes and their potential for causing injuries, with subsequent risk reduction systems being put in place. Hence, the introduction of the requirement for carrying out *risk assessments*.

The legal framework relating to health and safety in the developed world has a common theme of a *duty of care*. This duty of care, and common consideration to do no harm, goes back to the Magna Carta, which was signed in 1215 at Runnymede, England. The access to a legal concept of being able to seek justice for wrongs that have been done is not only the basis of common law in the UK, but also has an influence on health and safety legislation, which requires people to work in a manner that reduces the risk of causing harm to others.

The legal system is made of two distinct areas. First, the statute law is governed by the laws and regulations that form the laws of the land. Secondly, the common law enables redress for wrongs or losses that one party has caused another. Statute law uses words such as 'will' and 'shall', which indicate that compliance is not optional. However, common law is based on judicial precedent, which means that previous judgments of past cases form the bases of future judgments. In simple terms, breaking statute laws can incur a criminal record, whereas civil claims through the use of common law are for compensation of a loss. Losses may be sustained for many reasons, such as pain from an injury or disability or stress caused by poorly managed working environments.

## The Working Environment

The modern veterinary practice presents a complex working environment, not only in the treatments that can be offered, but also the range of equipment that is available. Equipment can range from electrically powered clippers for the removal of fur, to lifting equipment in the equine practice, to chemical hazards such as the handling of cytotoxic drugs used in the treatment of cancers.

When considering the work environment we need to think about how the environment determines the different ways of working, which in turn can influence how we manage treatments for the patients. Within this environment, issues such as the ergonomics of various tasks and how these tasks are carried out will influence the outcome of a patient's treatment. The environment itself and the treatment regimes may have an effect on the health and safety of those carrying out treatments. It can also be argued that the availability of facilities and the opportunity for staff to take breaks to eat and drink can influence the outcome of treatments as well, in that staff who are tired, hungry or thirsty will not be able to give their best attention to patients. Tired staff are also more likely to make mistakes that can result in a colleague or client being injured.

## The 'Risk Assessment' Concept

The concept of the '*risk assessment*' has been used by man as a survival tool since prehistoric times when hunters had to weigh up the likelihood of the animal that they were hunting for food turning on them and killing them instead. Formalizing a risk reduction strategy is useful, because when all the elements of the task are fully considered, improvements can be made. A risk assessment enables us to think about the *potential for harm*, that is, the potential severity of an injury, as well as the *frequency* of the undertaking of a particular task. It is important to also consider whether there is, in fact, a better or 'less risky' method of doing a task: one that by a simple substitution of one chemical for another or by devising a different way of working, for example, can reduce the likelihood of an injury and the severity of any potential injury. Although this would be the ideal situation, clearly our patients will not have grasped the concept of risk assessment. They have a free will, which may be expressed as defensive behaviour in response to an unfamiliar environment or, perhaps, to inadequate analgesia following surgery when they may exhibit what appears to be aggression, but may instead be motivated by discomfort and self-defence. In this kind of situation, it is almost impossible to write a risk assessment to cover every eventuality. Therefore, the concept of a *dynamic risk assessment* is useful.

## The 'Dynamic Risk Assessment' Concept

The dynamic risk assessment is simply a risk assessment made on the spot at the time of the activity where there is an element of unpredictability. If a patient needs to be assessed following surgery, this involves handling the patient but, before handling, there needs to be careful observation of the patient with regard to noise, or any other cause of stress. This is where clinical experience is required, not just academic knowledge. We need to be able to 'read' a patient's posture and actions, with and without our interaction. We need to consider clinical evidence, such as the analgesia provided to a patient post surgery, or whether the patient has been in one position on an operating table for any length of time, which may have caused postural discomfort.

Risk assessments also need to consider when a task is carried out. If we are treating a patient at the surgery at night, there will be fewer staff than during the day, which means fewer people to help move or treat a patient, which may lead to the patient not being handled in the most appropriate way, resulting in the patient becoming defensive.

## Home Visit Considerations

The planning process for any visit away from the normal working environment should consider not only how best to care for the patient, but how to ensure the health and safety of the staff so that the necessary care can be given to the patient effectively.

We may be carrying drugs that have the potential for abuse, or we may be going to an unfamiliar location, requiring discretion to reduce the attention we draw to ourselves.

There are a number of additional considerations:

- How many staff should attend?
- What is the availability of escape routes (for the pet and for us!)?
- Does someone else know where we are?
- What time are expected to return to the practice?

- Is the patient guarding the home or the owner (or both) and exhibiting different behaviour to that seen in the practice environment where they may have been subdued?

These may start off as unanswered questions, but by looking at the worst-case scenario we can prepare a plan before making a home visit. One area that is often overlooked is access to a suitable place to examine the patient. This should ideally be somewhere that provides a good escape route in case the patient becomes defensive. Additionally, consideration needs to be given to the ability of the owner to assist in any examination that is required.

A risk assessment for home visits will also include consideration of any equipment needed to enable a patient to be examined or safely transferred to the practice environment for continued treatment. Such equipment may include muzzles or carry cages.

## Risks Associated with Specific Areas and Work Practices

Within the practice environment, specific areas, work practices and equipment may present a risk. The aim is to reduce this risk so that it is as low as is practicably possible. The specific risks we can encounter are cytotoxic drugs, electrical equipment (which may need to be used in an environment where there is water present), manual handling of the patients as well as the handling and storage of items such as pet food. Involvement in equine or farm animal practice will carry additional risks associated with lifting equipment such as winches, hoists or lifting platforms. The presence of pressure systems is also an area to consider as the modern practice will house gas cylinders, anaesthetic machines, autoclaves and dental equipment powered by compressed air, among others, all of which require specific considerations pertinent to the risks associated with them.

The risks from explosions and fires associated with anaesthesia and surgery are greatly reduced compared with a few decades ago, when flammable and volatile anaesthetic agents were the norm, but there is still a risk from some sterilization methods, such as in the use of ethylene oxide, which is highly flammable or explosive under certain circumstances. Due care is needed and a safe system of working should be formulated, following a risk assessment, to ensure there is adequate provision for venting the used ethylene oxide and a reduction of sources of ignition in the vicinity of the ethylene oxide sterilizer. Where fire is concerned, the liberal use of spirit-based skin disinfectants has the potential to provide a fuel vapour. In conjunction with an ignition source from surgical diathermy, there is a real risk of fire, which will injure the patient and potentially also any staff in the immediate vicinity. Add to this an oxygen-rich environment, and the potential for *serious* injury to staff, as well as to the patient, increases significantly. Spirit fires in operating theatres have caused burns that have resulted in the death of a patient and severe burns to staff.

## Chemicals

In any practice environment there will be chemicals, whether these are domestic in nature, such as cleaning materials, or drugs or specialist cleaning solutions. All the chemicals used have the potential to cause harm, even humble washing-up liquid may cause an allergic reaction in some people due to its constituents, such as perfumes or limonenes used for degreasing. Degreasing surfaces to remove biological contamination may be good for the clinical environment, but degreasing skin leaves it prone to infection as the skin cracks, so the regular use of detergents should be considered as potentially hazardous. Care of the skin is very important. Occupational dermatitis is one of the major causes of industrial injury in the workplace (along with slips, trips and falls). Some medicines need careful handling to prevent adverse reactions from inhalation, ingestion or percutaneous absorption. Reading the safety data sheets from the manufacturers will give advice on handling and managing spillages. The data sheets are available free of charge from the suppliers, which have a legal responsibility to provide this information.

Understanding the nature of the chemical compound and any risks associated with mixing the compound with another should be considered in an assessment of the handling, use and disposal of any chemical used in the practice. If the chemical compound has been assessed as relatively safe for routine use, it is worth recording this fact. However, if the chemical compound is assessed to have a significant risk factor, it is prudent to consider replacing it with a safer alternative rather than introducing protective measures, such as personal protective equipment.

## Sharps

The handling of sharps and the potential for injuries, whether cuts or needle-stick injuries, should be considered within the framework of good practice in the clinical environment. The potential for harm from a relatively small initial injury needs to be considered and the good management of sharps not only protects the person using the sharp, but also others in the clinical environment. Good handling techniques are learned from experienced staff with good clinical skills. If there are junior staff undergoing training, it is worth noting that blank blades are available from the scalpel blade manufacturers for practising handling techniques (Fig. 12.1a, b, c).

(a)

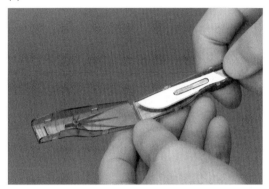

(b)

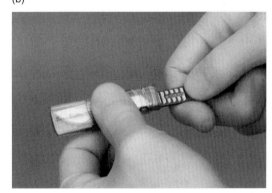

(c)

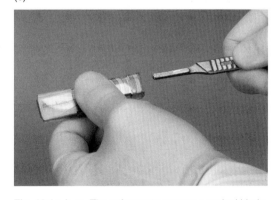

**Fig. 12.1a, b, c.** The safe way to remove a scalpel blade.

## Radiation

Radiation from X-ray machines or isotopes needs to be considered within the legal framework of the country that they are being used in. Specific guidance and legislation are usually available from learned professional societies.

## Management and Staff Cooperation

There is a legal requirement for managers to consult staff on changes to the health and safety management of an organization. This is usually through a union safety representative or by open meetings. The significant part of this requirement is the exchange of information between the management and staff in both directions. A benefit of this is that all those in the practice take some ownership of the health and safety in the practice.

## Useful Sources of Information

UK legislation and legal guidance on implementation of the law is available online from the following government organizations:

The Official Home of UK Legislation. Available at: www. legislation.gov.uk (accessed 5 June 2012).

Health and Safety Executive, UK. Available at: www.hse. gov.uk (accessed 5 June 2012).

Health Protection Agency, UK. Available at: www.hpa. org.uk (accessed 5 June 2012).

Environment Agency, UK. Available at: www.environment-agency.gov.uk (accessed 5 June 2012).

Also, consider contacting your trade union for advice.

# 13 Managing Health and Safety in a Clinical Environment

ALAN JONES

Health and safety management is a responsibility that should not be undertaken without appropriate training. When undertaking such duties for the first time in veterinary practice, it is advisable to obtain the guidance of a qualified health and safety professional. There are many different hazards in a veterinary practice, which must be appropriately managed. Responsibility for health and safety lies with the business owner, who may delegate management duties relating to health and safety to others. This chapter aims to discuss the most important hazards and their associated risks, and to explain how these should be effectively managed to ensure the safety of all staff, clients and visitors.

## Anaesthetic Waste Gas Scavenging

Anaesthetic waste gas scavenging is the safe removal of volatile and gaseous anaesthetic agents once they have been exhaled from a patient during anaesthesia. The systems used can be active or passive, but aim to produce the same result.

Active systems rely on a fan to move the diluted exhaled gas away from the patient and then discharge the mixed gases to the outside of the building. In these active systems, the fan is positioned remotely from the patient and an air break is incorporated between the breathing system and the fan to prevent a negative pressure being exerted on the breathing system. The air break is usually designed on the principle of one tube inside another, with the outer tube connected to the fan unit and the inner tube connected to the breathing system expiratory valve. The patient breathes out, pushing the exhaled gas into the gas flow created by the fan unit. The benefit of this system is that the patient only has the resistance of a short length of tubing distal to the expiratory valve. The diluted gas mixture is then discharged outside the building in a way that minimizes the chance of the expelled gas mixture from re-entering the building through open doors or windows (Fig. 13.1a, b)

Passive systems use the patient's expiratory efforts to move expired gases to the exterior of the practice building. An alternative passive method uses an absorbent canister to remove organic volatile compounds (VOCs) from the exhaled gas (Fig. 13.2). This absorber system has a distinct disadvantage in that nitrous oxide is not absorbed by the activated charcoal. In some designs of operating theatre, passive systems are used that utilize the inherent air flow for the air exchanges, but these systems are no longer seen in new buildings.

To determine whether the scavenging systems and protocols are being used properly, environmental contamination can be measured using either a system for monitoring the gross environment, which usually involves the employment of a mass spectrometer, or one that requires staff to wear personal dosimeters. The latter option is the preferred option for small and large practices, as the doses recorded are closely linked to the activities of individuals. Results using this method are usually expressed as parts per million averaged over the equivalent of an 8 hour period. This system of calculation is usually referred to as a time weighted average (TWA). An example may be read as 0.9 ppm isoflurane TWA. Each volatile agent and nitrous oxide will have its own limit given as a TWA, and these will have different values. As a general rule, it is best to ensure that personal exposures are within 50% of the TWA for any agent. However, in practice, if all the systems are working well, the results should be within 10% of the TWA. Any increase seen in the regular environmental monitoring results should be investigated, as this may indicate that a part of the scavenging system is in need of servicing or that procedures are not being followed.

Each country has its own standards, which can usually be sourced via a Web search using the name of the volatile agent and 'occupational exposure' as search terms.

© C.R. Coates 2012. *Veterinary Practice Management* (C.R. Coates)

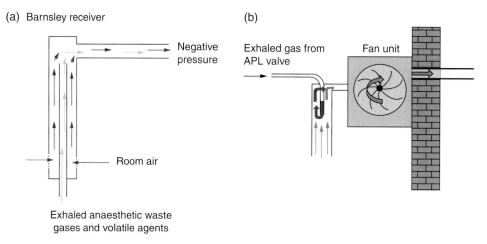

(a) Barnsley receiver

Negative pressure

Room air

Exhaled anaesthetic waste
gases and volatile agents

(b)

Exhaled gas from
APL valve

Fan unit

**Fig. 13.1.** Anaesthetic waste gas active scavenging. (a) This part of the system entrains the room air to dilute the exhaled anaesthetic agents. The device shown is called a Barnsley receiver. The darker arrow represents room air and the paler arrow represents the exhaled anaesthetic waste from the patient. (b) The wall fan arrangement for active scavenging, which applies negative pressure to the Barnsley receiver outlet. APL valve, adjustable pressure-limiting valve.

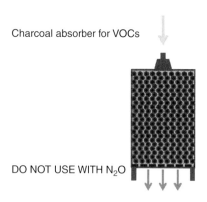

Charcoal absorber for VOCs

DO NOT USE WITH $N_2O$

**Fig. 13.2.** Passive anaesthetic waste gas scavenging. The absorber contains activated charcoal that absorbs volatile organic compounds (VOCs), such as isoflurane, from the exhaled gases. This absorber does not absorb nitrous oxide. The downward arrow illustrates the flow of gas from the patient's anaesthetic breathing system.

## Control of Hazardous Chemicals

### Drugs

Cytotoxic drugs, by the nature of their actions, are inherently toxic and handling of these drugs carries its own risks to the staff who are administering them. There is usually specific guidance from national organizations that produce information on the correct storage, handling and administration of such drugs. Advisory guidelines also provide information on the correct disposal procedure for the drugs and any associated animal excretions or exudates that may be contaminated with unchanged drug or with physiologically active metabolites.

Reconstituting cytotoxic drugs for intravenous administration is best carried out in the confines of a glove box with negative pressure and filters to absorb any mist or aerosol created when adding water to a vial of the dried drug in order to reconstitute it. If a glove box is not available, the risk of contamination to the person reconstituting the drug increases many fold, because there is less protection from potential aerosol or skin contamination. Gloves, disposable aprons, face masks and eye protection do not offer sufficient protection.

Some hormone preparations are absorbed through the skin, so the manner in which they are handled is very important. Although hormone preparations are used frequently in farm animal practice, there are still sufficient risks from handling these preparations in small animal practice. The risk assessment for handling the drugs should consider possible routes of personal contamination, the method of administration to the patient and the environment in which the person administering the drug is working. Consideration also needs to be given as to whether the person handling the drug is pregnant as some hormone preparations used to induce oestrus can also cause abortion in people. The risk assessment needs to consider not just the basic precautions, but also who is handling the drug.

## Cleaning chemicals

Bleach, acid cleaners, surface disinfectants and skin preparation solutions all have the potential to cause harm by inhalation, ingestion, and skin and mucosal contact. For this reason, chemical solutions, whether 'domestic' or clinical in use, should all be considered harmful until proved otherwise. Currently available cleaning chemicals will come with accompanying hazard data sheets from the manufacturers. These data sheets contain information on the constituents of the formulation, the potential for harm from chemical burns, skin absorption or the inhalation of vapour. There is also written information on the container itself specifying which other chemicals should not be used in conjunction with the chemical. An example of an inappropriate mixture is given by the hypochlorite bleach commonly used as a toilet bleach cleaner or surface disinfectant, and acid (descaling) toilet cleaners that claim to remove limescale. Mixing the acid toilet cleaner with bleach will produce chlorine gas, which is damaging to the mucous membranes, particularly the eyes and respiratory tract. A risk assessment under the Control of Substances Hazardous to Health (COSHH) regulations would highlight this unwanted reaction between the two toilet cleaners, make it plain that they should never be mixed and also that both the hypochlorite and acid cleaner are capable of causing significant skin damage if splashes are not washed off immediately.

Some surface disinfectants used in clinical environments are stated as being relatively safe when in contact with skin for short periods, but there are usually other ingredients added to these compounds that add a fragrance; these may contain limonenes, which are a powerful degreasant, disrupt the protective layer of the dermis and can lead to a reaction, such as occupational eczema. It is, therefore, important when assessing chemicals used in the practice to include information on all the constituents and not just the active ingredients.

## Ergonomics

The ergonomics of the work environment, both reception/office areas and clinical areas, need to be assessed for potential hazards. Some areas, where the potential for injury is not apparent immediately, may be overlooked during this assessment. Take, for example, the reception area. Transferring archive boxes of papers to the store room, handling heavy bags of prescription diets, moving between the computer screen and the telephone are common activities, representing a considerable amount of movement and manual handling that could lead to injuries, particularly if the movements are repetitive. Also, it should be remembered that being in one position for too long can cause physical problems, such as joint stiffness and poor circulation to the lower extremities. A good mix of supported sitting posture and other activities requiring standing and moving are the way forward to reduce musculoskeletal injuries.

Computer workstations should be adjustable so that different users can configure the chairs to suit their own height, with screens adjustable for height and angle of view to reduce the risk of poor neck posture and eliminate glare and other distractions, which may cause unusual posture and lead to headaches. If a lot of data entry is required from typed or handwritten sheets, then the provision of a copy stand may prove useful; this will allow the neck to be kept at a normal posture with some movement to reduce stiffness. The lighting should not reflect off the screen or shiny surfaces, as this could cause eye strain. Even relatively simple items of office equipment have been implicated in injuries at work, such as the paper shredder, which can trap loose clothing, hair or fingers, resulting in serious injury.

The incidence of work-related upper limb disorder (previously referred to as repetitive strain injury or RSI) remains a cause for concern. However, the number of reported incidents is reducing, as the causes and remedial actions required to eliminate them are becoming better known in the workplace. Complacency over this type of work-related injury is not an option though, and constant vigilance is required to ensure continuity of a safe working environment. Work-related upper limb disorder (WRULD) also includes neck strain, which may lead to headaches. The problem with these disorders is that they take a long time to improve and may require significant input from a physiotherapist to resolve.

Nursing staff may have been taught how to lift safely, but as the reception area is usually the place where deliveries are received, it makes sense to ensure that receptionists are also taught this. If goods need to be lifted off high shelves, steps of an approved design should be used, but then the issue may arise of whether the activity of stocking and dispensing from high shelves is classified as 'working at height', which has its own set of regulations, rules and guidance. A better solution is not to use shelves that require steps to reach them and to consider the weights of items put on high shelves. The UK Health and Safety Executive has very good guidance on this matter, which is free to download from its web site.

The general working environment should be warm enough to be comfortable in the clothing normally worn at work. Lighting should be sufficiently bright to enable normal tasks to be carried out safely without eye strain, but not too bright so as to cause headaches or excessive glare. Toilet, washing and rest facilities are also a necessity, as well as allowing staff to have regular rest breaks away from the working environment. These issues are covered in the welfare regulations that form part of health and safety legislation.

## Electrical Equipment

Legislation requires that electrical equipment is regularly tested to ensure that it is safe to use. The timing of this formal testing is determined by a risk assessment that takes into account how often the equipment is used and the environment in which it is used. Other factors should also be considered, such as, for example, whether the equipment is frequently moved from place to place. Take two different items – clippers and computers. These two items vary in their risks. The clippers could be dropped, the cable may be strained or the insulation may be damaged. These types of common risk should lead us to ensure that we carry out routine visual inspections of all clippers before we plug them in to the mains supply. The computer, conversely, will rarely, if ever, be moved, and because it is subject to a much less rigorous life, it could reasonably be formally inspected and tested on a 3 year cycle. The clippers, in contrast, need to be tested much more frequently – at least annually and, ideally, 6 monthly or even more frequently (Fig. 13.3).

Records must be kept of the testing that is formally carried out, all defects must be rectified and the equipment retested before the equipment is put back into service.

## Lifting Equipment

Lifting equipment can take many forms, from hoists to lift equine and farm animals from the anaesthetic induction box to the operating table, winches for moving patients inside the induction box and hydraulic platform operating tables. Each type of

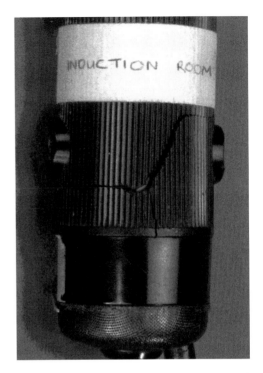

**Fig. 13.3.** Electrical clippers that have been dropped and are cracked. Although still capable of working, they present a significant risk of electrocution if they are used with the metal inside exposed.

lifting equipment has its own benefits when considering the alternative of moving a heavy animal manually. However, the use of any lifting equipment requires staff to be trained in its correct use and in the inherent risks associated with moving safely what is, perhaps, more than a tonne in weight of anaesthetized animal. The safe use of lifting equipment relies on appropriate instruction, supervision and training, and sufficient information being supplied to persons using the equipment. A record of the training should be made and regularly updated.

Lifting equipment must be regularly inspected to check that it is working correctly and to detect any wear in chains, cables or hydraulic seals. The best time to do this is before the equipment is going to be used and before the induction of anaesthesia. In addition to these pre-use checks, there are legal requirements for the regular inspection, servicing and maintenance of lifting equipment by a competent person. A competent person is usually defined as someone with specialist knowledge of the type of lifting equipment concerned. Inspections and maintenance are carried out within the framework of a written scheme of examination that ensures all the functions and parts subject to wear are thoroughly inspected with remedial actions taken or advised, depending on the type of inspection. Most countries have statutory inspections that are required by law, so it is imperative that these are arranged on a timely basis. Legislation also requires that additional equipment used for lifting operations is marked with the safe working load and a traceable number to ensure that it is suitable for the purpose for which it was designed (Figs 13.4, 13.5 and 13.6).

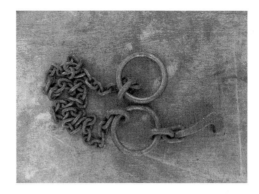

**Fig. 13.6.** This lifting chain is *unsafe* to use as it has no safe working load marked.

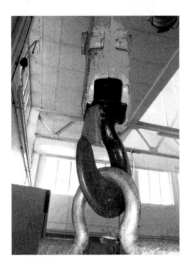

**Fig. 13.4.** Lifting equipment hook showing safety catch in place.

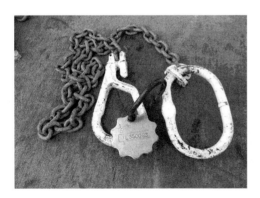

**Fig. 13.5.** Lifting chain showing safe working load, which is stamped on the identifying disc in kilos, along with a serial number for identification purposes. It is important that the disc is present and is permanently attached, showing that the equipment is safe to use, as here.

Older methods of manufacture of hobbles for lifting horses on to and off operating tables utilizing, for example, leather, are not acceptable in modern practice, as the leather will vary in strength between the batches made and only destruction testing will satisfy the requirements of ascertaining a safe working load; this would, unfortunately, destroy the hobble in the process. Modern hobbles that are made of reproducible modern synthetic materials lead to consistency and does allow for batch testing of the nylon webbing used and a safe working load indication to be applied to the ancillary equipment. A sample of the finished hobbles will be tested to the safe working load plus a percentage, to ensure the hobbles do not break under the specified safe working load. All lifting equipment must be identifiable and clearly marked with the safe working load, which must not be exceeded. All lifting accessories such as slings (including hobbles) have a finite working life, which also must not be exceeded.

## Pressure Systems

Pressure systems within the veterinary practice will include autoclaves for the sterilization of surgical instruments, medical gas pipelines, anaesthetic machines, medical/surgical air plants and pressure receivers for dental equipment. All these types of equipment require regular inspection by a suitable person, usually defined as someone with appropriate qualifications and experience in the type of equipment concerned.

Pressure systems have stored energy in the form of compressed gas, or in the case of an autoclave, steam. This stored energy must not be released in such a way that it can cause injury. Therefore, safety features built in to the equipment require regular inspections that comply with a written scheme of examination, both for inspection and servicing. The written scheme lists the functions to be tested and areas to be inspected to ensure normal safe functioning.

Typical features that are tested include safety valves that release excess pressure safely in a controlled manner and the condition of seals that contain the pressure and the functional operation of the equipment. Routine replacement of seals with a known life expectancy is undertaken during the servicing of the equipment.

Patient safety considerations also need to be taken into account, such as when the medical gas pipeline system is changed, modified or adapted. In these circumstances, the medical gas pipeline system is checked by a specially trained pharmacist to avoid confusion between the outlets, and to check purity of the gas, and particulate and moisture contents. This type of check is only required if the pipeline system has been cut and rejoined to change its configuration, perhaps for the addition of extra wall outlets as the practice expands.

When installing a medical gas pipeline system it is prudent to ensure that isolation valves are strategically placed within the system which will allow for routine maintenance while the system is pressurized and also for the shutting off of gas to an area of the building if a general fire occurs. Ideally, one of the valves should be positioned so that all the gas to the building can be cut off. These isolation valves are behind break glass enclosures so that all staff have access to the valves in case of an emergency. For servicing there is usually key access to the valves.

With any pressurized gas system no oil or grease must come into contact with any part of the system. Fires have been recorded where a small gas leak has ignited grease or oil that has been left on the pipework or seals. Fires caused by the release of compressed gas can be fierce enough to melt metal and can be a real threat to life of staff and patients. There are anecdotal reports of fires being started by a person changing an oxygen cylinder after using hand lotion. The hand lotion contained sufficient grease for a small oxygen leak from between the cylinder valve and a cylinder yoke to be sufficient to cause ignition, with subsequent damage to the cylinder yoke.

## Animal Handling

Animals by nature have free will and so we cannot with absolute certainty say that an animal will behave in a predictable manner every time that it is handled. Well-behaved animals that allow handling are submitting their choice to follow the owner's instructions to possibly please the owner, but there is always a possibility that the animal may react in an adverse way. Most people who work with particular species regularly will be able to read body language from members of that species, but even they cannot say with absolute certainty that they can read all members of a species all of the time. Animals can be defensive when in unfamiliar environments that they perceive as threatening. Hence, dynamic risk assessments for animal handling, as well as formal risk assessments that consider issues such as manual handling and zoonotic infection risks, should be carried out. A simple tool for reducing the risk of zoonotic disease transmission is hand washing; this can often be overlooked with the time pressures resulting from a heavy workload. However, good personal hygiene is vital to reducing cross-infection between patients, as well as the spread of disease to humans. It is always worth making time for good hand washing.

There are many good textbooks and institutional teaching that include sound animal handling principles, but there is no substitute for experience and being able to read the animal's behaviour. Learning about animal behaviour so that new animal care staff are equipped to work safely with animals requires information, instruction, training and supervision. Suitable and sufficient staff training is a legal requirement under health and safety statutes and must, therefore, be provided. It is also prudent to record training, such as the type of training provided and undertaken, the date it was undertaken and, possibly, some form of assessment, if this is considered necessary. Not all staff will have the necessary skills to handle all species, so it is worth noting if a particular member of staff is particularly good with a specific species or not so proficient with a species. It is also worth noting that many owners are not proficient at handling their animals, especially if the animals are stressed in a clinical environment. It is, consequently, prudent not to ask the owner to hold the patient for examination or treatment. The person in charge of the procedure has a duty of care to those in the vicinity, which includes the owners, who may also be at risk.

## Manual Handling of Animals

Courses are available in manual handling and these provide a good basis for assessing the manual handling protocols that are followed in the practice. However, many of these courses are primarily concerned with the lifting and moving of boxes and other regular-shaped articles. Handling patients is complicated by the patients, because they are not regular in shape, they have many different sizes, conformities and weights and move of their own free will. Therefore, a different approach to manual handling is required. Primarily, the principles of good lifting posture and the use of additional manpower need to be considered, not just because of the weight of the patient, but also because of the flexibility of a body that can shift its centre of gravity during a lift, thus causing injury to the person or persons doing the lifting.

Any anxiety that the patient experiences during a manual handling procedure may cause an adverse defensive reaction, such as biting or struggling to get free. With patient lifting, it is realistic to reduce the suggested safe lifting limits. Consideration also needs to be given to the potential for doing harm to the patient during a manual handling procedure, so the interests of the patient as well as the persons doing the lifting should be considered together.

Planning is a key part of moving patients. This planning should be done before the lifting/handling procedure. In every case it should be understood what each person's role is and who is in charge of the timing of the procedure. Traditionally, the person in control of the animal's head is the person who dictates when a lift of a patient can be carried out. The person controlling the head is also working to ensure the patient is not in a position to bite those lifting the patient. That person must also make sure that everyone involved in the lift is ready and in position before the lift is started.

## Fire and First Aid

Planning for fire or some other hazard that may require evacuation from the practice is a legal requirement. A safe place needs to be identified and indicated as an assembly point, with staff being allocated specific tasks, such as checking that the building is clear by a roll call or sweep of the building (if there is no immediate risk to the person carrying out the sweep).

Should patients be evacuated during a fire is a question that is often asked. If the building needs to be evacuated, it is not, by definition, safe to attempt to remove patients from kennels. The fire doors fitted should offer some protection from smoke

inhalation if expansion strips have been fitted and the doors are of a suitable fire-resistant construction to enable the rescue services to rescue the patients. Putting human life at risk is not an option. Taking a patient already on a lead with you to the assembly point is acceptable. Current building regulations and fire precautions should offer sufficient protection for a rescue to be effected by the fire and rescue service. It should go without saying that wedging fire doors open is dangerous and illegal and could result in prosecution of the individual and the organization.

The fire risk assessment should cover the actions to be taken by staff during a fire and should include the responsibilities of individuals, such as reception staff, being responsible for evacuating the clients and their pets to the assembly point. Another member of staff may be required to shut off any oxygen feed to the building. These responsibilities should be detailed in the fire risk assessment and all staff should know their duties during an evacuation. A fire risk assessment should also specify the frequency of any fire evacuation drills, call-point testing and maintenance of any fire alarm system in place.

As there is potential for injuries from the work environment and possibly from an adverse reaction from a patient, every practice must have in place a first aid procedure. Specific training is advisable for first aiders. Although many in medical or veterinary professions feel they are adequately qualified to administer first aid, there are considerations other than dressing a wound, such as the management of an incident and proper reporting systems for injuries. It is, therefore, essential that a suitable number of people are trained in first aid and that they are numerous enough to ensure that someone is always available to provide first aid when needed. There is specific legislation concerning fire safety and first aid requirements in a work undertaking. These requirements are covered by statute law and, consequently, must be followed.

## Accidents

It is a legal requirement to maintain a record of accidents that occur in the workplace. These records are required to be presented in the event of a civil law claim against the practice for damages that result from an accident. There is a specific requirement that accidents which result in certain injuries, such as fractures to long bones, head injuries and injuries that cause prolonged absence from work, are reported to the UK Health and Safety Executive (HSE). The specific details are contained in the first aid regulations. Advice can be obtained from the HSE. Included in these regulations are occupational illness and work-related diseases, such as dermatitis, asthma and notifiable diseases. The Reporting of Injuries, Diseases and Dangerous Occurrences Regulations (RIDDOR) is the primary legislation in the UK covering work-related injuries, disability and illness caused by work.

## Pregnancy

The pregnant person must inform the practice manager of the pregnancy in writing. This is a requirement before any risk assessment is undertaken. The manager has the right to ask for the pregnancy to be confirmed by a registered midwife or a medical practitioner. Failure to comply with written notification of the pregnancy removes the requirement for the risk assessment and subsequent work changes that may be necessary. It is advisable to read the specific guidance from health and safety bodies, such as the HSE.

Following formal notification by the pregnant employee, the manager will arrange a meeting with to discuss future work and the working environment. The risk assessment for the pregnancy is specific to the individual employee and the work that the employee undertakes. It is also worth mentioning that *all* health and safety risks need to be considered, including mental health risks, such as stress in the workplace.

To ensure the health and safety of pregnant employees, specific precautions must be taken. First, the tasks undertaken by any pregnant persons as part of their job need to undergo a risk assessment. This risk assessment must be specific to their role and must also include consideration of working hours and the working environment. The working environment may have included time spent in locations where X-rays are used, in cat accommodation, or handling hormones or cytotoxic drugs. These will have to be excluded from future work. Night-time working may have an adverse effect on the pregnant person's well-being and this may well need to cease, as may any 'on call' duties, both for the duration of the pregnancy and in the period following the birth.

The risk assessment carried out must be specific to the person concerned, as there may be differences in working conditions of people of a similar grade or in similar professions. The specific risks that the individual is exposed to need to be listed and used as a framework for the risk assessment, with each of the risks addressed separately. Risk reduction may not be an option for some of these risks. Therefore, risk avoidance is the practical way forward, for example, not being in the room when X-rays are being taken or ensuring that anaesthetic gas scavenging is working to the best of its ability. Personal dose monitoring may be required to quantify any potential environmental contamination. It is prudent to remove the pregnant person from this environment until there is confirmation that the scavenging is adequate.

Psychological aspects to the risk assessment should also be considered. It is not unusual for pregnant persons to be very worried about a work undertaking, so if there is the potential for them to feel stress about an aspect of the work adversely affecting the pregnancy, it is worth ensuring that they do not come into contact with that area of the practice. Although this may seem unnecessary, it is looking after the mental health of the pregnant person, which is the practice owner's responsibility.

## Waste

Waste produced by the practice is classified into a number of different types: domestic, industrial, clinical and special. Segregation of the waste at source is important as the handling methods used for the different categories of waste are different. Domestic waste equivalent to household rubbish will be classified as industrial waste, as it comes from a business and, consequently, needs to be treated as such.

Clinical waste contains items that are likely to be contaminated by blood, tissue or other body fluids which may carry harmful bacteria. Special waste usually consists of waste that is contaminated by cytotoxic drugs or harmful pathogens. Full descriptions of waste management and disposal can be found on the Internet for the specific country. Usually, waste management comes under separate legislation to health and safety statutes. However, any failure to comply with waste management requirements that causes, or could cause, injury could be subject to the failure of a duty of care under health and safety legislation as well as have the potential to be prosecuted under environmental legislation. It is the duty of the business undertaking to ensure that any waste produced by it is disposed of in accordance with the relevant legislation. Reputable specialist waste carriers are the preferred choice for handling clinical waste and special waste. In the UK, the person producing the waste is responsible for ensuring that the waste is dealt with appropriately by the contractor. It is, therefore, prudent to ensure that the contractor is able to demonstrate an audit trail of the carriage and final destruction of the waste.

## CE Marking

In the European Union (EU) items for sale are marked with a CE label, which indicates that the item conforms to the minimum standards required for sale and distribution, but if a practice imports items from outside the EU, the practice itself is responsible for ensuring that these standards are met by the item that has been imported. If the only source of a piece of equipment is a supplier in a country outside the EU, then the importer must ensure the item is fit for purpose and complies with the relevant specifications. If an item is ordered directly from the manufacturers, it is prudent to ensure that the manufacturer can state that the item complies with the relevant specifications. Alternatively, the order for the equipment could be placed through an agent who will be obliged to ensure compliance. The onus is on the practice to ensure that goods purchased comply with the required standards. Equipment from other countries may be of a suitable standard or even exceed that required, but the CE mark is the definitive indicator of compliance with European standards.

## Workplace Stress

Every workplace has some moments of stress, but if the stress is affecting a person's health and well-being, it must be managed and changes made to reduce the stress. The mental health of staff needs to be considered as well as their physical health. Useful information on this topic is available from the HSE web site. Workplace stress and management failure to address the issues involved have led to significant awards in the civil courts against the companies, businesses and organizations that have failed to address the problems. Time and effort reducing stress in the workplace is cost-effective.

## Communication

A good workplace has an open safety culture where the staff and management are able to discuss safety issues freely. From a management perspective, a safe workplace is also more productive with less time lost through sickness, injury or stress.

## Useful Sources of Information

UK legislation and legal guidance on implementation of the law is available online from the following government organizations:

The Official Home of UK Legislation. Available at: www.legislation.gov.uk (accessed 5 June 2012).

Health and Safety Executive, UK. Available at: www.hse.gov.uk (accessed 5 June 2012).

Health Protection Agency, UK. Available at: www.hpa.org.uk (accessed 5 June 2012).

Environment Agency, UK. Available at: www.environment-agency.gov.uk (accessed 5 June 2012).

Also consider contacting your trade union for advice.

## Revision Questions

1. If you have not done so already, spend time familiarizing yourself with your practice's health and safety protocols. Is the available information complete and up to date?
2. Access the HSE web site and review the guidance there about workplace stress. Identify specific workplace stressors that exist for you and the ways in which you personally manage these.
3. Review the health and safety training that you have received and assess whether this is adequate for your needs. If not, take appropriate action.
4. Carry out a risk assessment of the reception area in your practice and produce a brief report of your findings, recommending specific actions that should be taken to improve the safety of this area.

# 14 Effective Stock Management

The purchase of drugs and medicines is the largest practice expense after staff salaries (Shilcock and Stutchfield, 2008). Of course, sales are correspondingly high. Macfarlane and Robson (2011) cite XLVets (a group of independently owned, progressive veterinary practices) key performance indicator data which suggest that medicines sales per veterinarian within the UK small animal veterinary sector amount to around £81,500 per annum. For farm animal veterinarians, the figure is around £147,000 and for equine veterinarians around £44,500 per annum. Clearly, the movement of stock into and out of a veterinary practice represents substantial sums of money spent and earned. Accordingly, at any one time, a practice will keep considerable stocks on the premises and these have to be managed appropriately and in accordance with existing legislation.

The purpose of this chapter is to outline the principles of an effective stock management system, which can be applied not only to the management of stocks of drugs and medicines intended for resale to clients, but also to stocks of consumables intended for use within the practice. Guidance on the specific procedures that must be followed under UK and EU veterinary medicines regulations is available from the Veterinary Medicines Directorate (VMD) and the British Small Animal Veterinary Association (BSAVA), among others. Although this guidance will be referred to in the chapter, it will not be discussed in any detail.

## Why Apply Good Stock Control?

There are many good reasons for implementing a sound stock control system:

- To meet the day-to-day needs of the veterinary practice – so that the right medicines are available when required in the correct quantities, and so that the practice does not run out of essential drugs and medicines which could be detrimental to the health and welfare of the animals under the practice's care and to the business as a whole.

- To keep practice costs down – wholesalers and suppliers are now able to provide a reliable, daily delivery service, which means that it is no longer necessary for practices to purchase or keep large quantities of stock (although greater discounts are available for bulk purchases and the practice, especially large animal practices, may wish to take advantage of these). An efficient stock control system includes effective ordering procedures which ensure that the necessary stocks are available and that over ordering is prevented. This means that cash is not tied up in stock unnecessarily and can be used elsewhere.

- To prevent wastage, losses and theft – an effective stock control system will ensure that stocks are used up before they go out of date, that all breakages or damage are recorded and explained and that medicines which cannot be used for legitimate reasons are disposed of correctly and recorded. A system which ensures that all stock movements are accounted for will also help to eliminate thefts or 'borrowing' of medicines for own use.

- To ensure compliance with legal requirements – for example, in the UK, the requirements of the Veterinary Medicines Regulations 2007 must be met by all practices. Under these regulations, practices are required to carry out regular audits of their stocks of veterinary medicinal products (VMPs) and have in place an effective stock control system which can demonstrate to inspectors of practice premises that all VMPs are accounted for at all times. VMPs are defined as all drugs and medicines intended for treating or preventing disease in animals or for restoring normal physiological functions.

© C.R. Coates 2012. *Veterinary Practice Management* (C.R. Coates)

# The Stock Control System

## System set-up

Accurate record keeping is the basis of any good stock control system. As a starting point, assuming that a computerized stock database is going to form the hub of any system, it is necessary to create the database and populate it with stock details. When such a database is being set up for the first time, someone has to enter the information manually. Modern practice management systems will already have a database of common drugs and medicines provided as part of the software package, but this will most certainly need amendment, with additions or deletions made to it before it can be utilized. Each stock record created should contain the following information:

- Name of the drug/medicine/consumable.
- Units – pack size (if a drug or medicine comes in different pack sizes, there will be several stock records for the same drug or medicine).
- Unique catalogue or supplier reference number.
- Location – i.e. where the stock item is stored in the practice, whether stock is normally held in several different locations.
- Current stock level – to match the quantities currently held on the practice shelves.
- Minimum stock level – the level below which the amount held in stock cannot fall.
- Maximum stock level – the amount held in stock should not exceed this level.
- Reorder level – worked out by taking the minimum stock level and adding the average daily issue of the item multiplied by the number of days it will take for the supplier to deliver. Once the stock of the particular item falls to this level, an order will be triggered.
- Unit cost to the practice.
- Markup percentage to be applied.
- Sales price (price to the client).

Once the database is set up, any additions to the stock must be entered manually or uploaded from a hand-held scanner. Any sales to clients via the computer system will automatically update the existing stock levels and inform the user when stocks need to be replenished once holdings reach the reorder level. Setting minimum, maximum and reorder levels will involve some guesswork at the start, but over time, as experience is gained and as knowledge of the practice's operations builds, it should be possible to set these levels more accurately. It is good

practice to review them periodically in any case, taking into account seasonal variations.

## Day-to-day management

### Movements in to and out of stock

All practice purchases of veterinary drugs and medicines should record the following information:

- The date received
- The practice's unique order number
- Description of the product
- Batch number
- The quantity received
- The name and address of the supplier
- Supplier's delivery note number.

When the drugs and medicines are then sold to clients, the above records should be 'completed' by entering the date the drug/medicine was issued, the quantity supplied, the case reference number or unique client number, the animal name and the name and address of the client. If a prescription was issued, the name and address of the person issuing the prescription should also be recorded (Vernon, 2008). The practice computer system, or a separate computerized system, should enable the recording of all of the above information, but it is essential for all personnel involved in entering data to do so accurately and in a consistent manner. The practice computer system should also be able to produce detailed history reports on stock movements throughout a specified period. This is extremely useful not only for audit purposes, but also when a product is recalled by the manufacturer, which would necessitate contacting the relevant clients.

### Other deductions from stock

From time to time, despite everyone's best efforts, some stock items may go out of date and there may be accidental breakages or damage. Vernon (2008) recommends setting up appropriately named non-chargeable clients on the computer system to record such events (e.g. Out of Date Stock, or Stock Wastage). Doing so will ensure that these stock losses are not missed or forgotten. Additional non-chargeable stock 'clients' can be set up for receipts of free of charge products from suppliers and for correcting errors. If the practice computer system is going to be relied upon as an accurate record of all stock movements for audit purposes, it is essential to ensure that these out of the ordinary events are accurately recorded. Otherwise, there will hardly be any point in having a computerized system.

### General stock management

Good stock rotation should be employed, newly arrived stock being placed at the back of the shelf with older stock at the front. Effort should be maintained to rationalize stock holdings. For example, it may not be necessary to hold a number of different brands of the same formulation of ear drops or antibiotic or of every type of rubber glove or bandage. Veterinarians in the practice should routinely inspect stocks with the aim of identifying where reductions can be made. Sales representatives can be very persuasive and veterinarians will naturally wish to try out new products, but in purchasing a new product, they should decide which existing product the new product will replace rather than adding the new product to existing stocks.

In large animal or equine practices, stock held in cars should be regularly checked by a member of support staff whose job could also involve organizing and topping up car supplies and recording changes in stock levels at least twice a week.

To prevent stock going out of date, it is important to carry out regular date checks. If stock is stored in various locations in the practice, including cars, suitable individuals can be allocated specific areas to carry out checks, which could remain their responsibility. Any stock that is within 1 month of its expiry date should be removed, recorded as out of date and disposed of appropriately. A date-checking schedule should be drawn up and signed off after each date-checking exercise (BSAVA, 2012).

The procurement, storage, use and disposal of anaesthetics, sedatives and drugs used for euthanasia (known as 'controlled drugs') is governed by specific legislation in the UK and practices are required to adhere to this strictly. The VMD issues guidance on controlled drugs, which can be downloaded from their web site (VMD, 2011).

## Stock Audits

Macfarlane and Robson (2011) recommend that full medicines audits should become a regular feature of stock management in every practice.

A medicines audit is not simply an annual, year-end stocktake. It involves not only counting current stock holdings and reconciling these with computerized and other records, but also reviewing the entire process of purchasing, storing, supplying, prescribing and dispensing, and all associated record keeping. In the UK, it is a legal requirement for practices to carry out an audit of their VMPs at least once a year. Stock also represents an asset which the practice owns, the value of which must be established at the end of each financial year for accounting purposes.

### The stocktake

All stockholdings should be counted manually. This task is made easier if the stock is well organized in its various locations or in the pharmacy, and if staff are given a printed checklist of items stored in that location before they start. All staff should follow the same protocols for counting tablets and measuring or estimating quantities of liquids and powders. Ideally, the stock count should be carried out at a quiet time or out of hours and completed within a day. The results should then be compared with the computerized data and any discrepancies investigated and resolved. In a well-run system, the results of the manual stocktake will agree with the data held on the computer or in other records. If the discrepancies are small or relatively insignificant, this is most likely due to operator error, but if the discrepancies are significant, then there is cause for concern and the stocktake may need to be carried out again, and all purchase and sales records carefully scrutinized to establish what has gone wrong. If the previous stocktake was carried out a year ago, there may be a large number of records to work through. Hence the argument for carrying out more frequent stocktakes or 'rolling stocktakes', where specific sections of stock are counted in between audits (Macfarlane and Robson, 2011).

### The audit

To check whether procedures and record-keeping systems work well, the following data and documentation are required:

- Opening stock levels as per the last stocktake undertaken
- Closing stock levels as per current stocktake

- Detailed purchase data – obtained from the practice's ordering system
- Detailed sales data – obtained from the practice computer system
- Out-of-date, damaged or wasted stock data – obtained from the practice computer system or other record-keeping system, as appropriate to the practice
- All paper-based records pertaining to stock – copies of orders, purchase invoices, sales invoices, controlled drugs record books, copies of prescriptions issued, etc.

It would be a prohibitively time-consuming task to trace the history of every single stock item from purchase through to sale or disposal, so to make the task easier, a randomly generated list of 20 or so items can be used. Each item should then be carefully tracked from order generation through to its final destination. All of the records associated with each stage of the process should be checked at the same time to ensure that legal requirements are met and that the system works. The test of the system is, of course, when the equation

Opening stock + purchases – sales/disposals = closing stock

results in the current stocktake figure for all items selected for audit. This type of audit can be carried out for specific groups of drugs or medicines on a rotational basis, if preferred; this is more manageable than a full audit.

## Conclusion

This chapter has outlined a generic approach to stock management and control but, clearly, there is no one best method. Practices will naturally adopt systems and processes to suit their own circumstances. Much of what is done in veterinary practices in the UK is governed by legislation, and standard operating procedures are set out by bodies, such as the VMD, whose job it is to implement and enforce the law. This has made the task of managing inventory much more transparent and accountable, but has also resulted in an unprecedented amount of record keeping being required.

Practice owners and managers are responsible for ensuring that their systems meet both legal requirements and the needs of the practice and its clients. Complex systems require well-trained staff, who are not only familiar with the entire range of stock held, but also appreciate the importance of having sound and efficient systems and procedures.

## References

British Small Animal Veterinary Association (2012) *BSAVA Guide to the Use of Veterinary Medicines.* British Small Animal Veterinary Association, Quedgeley, UK. Available at: http://www.bsava.com (accessed 22 August 2011).

Macfarlane, J. and Robson, R. (2011) Counting your losses: medicines audits in practice. *In Practice* 33, 358–361.

Shilcock, M. and Stutchfield, G. (2008) *Veterinary Practice Management: A Practical Guide*, 2nd edn. Saunders Elsevier, Edinburgh, UK.

Vernon, R. (2008) Taking stock: ensuring accurate medicines records. *In Practice* 30, 582–583.

VMD (2011) *Controlled Drugs.* Veterinary Medicines Guidance Note 20. Veterinary Medicines Directorate, New Haw, UK. Available at http://www.vmd.defra.gov.uk/pdf/vmgn/VMGNote20.pdf (accessed 5 June 2012).

## Revision Questions

**1.** Familiarize yourself with the stock control procedures applicable in your practice. How closely do the procedures and record-keeping systems fit with those outlined in this chapter? Explain the reasons for the differences.

**2.** Access online the VMD Guidance Note entitled '*Controlled Drugs*'. Produce a summary, in your own words, of the record-keeping requirements, as outlined in this Guidance.

**3.** Produce a standard operating procedure (SOP) for dealing with a manufacturer's batch recall notice.

**4.** Familiarize yourself with the layout of the practice's pharmacy (or stock room) and ascertain the system that is used for organizing the items on the shelves. Is the layout logical, practical and convenient for staff? Are there any improvements that could be made?

# 15 Managing Computer Systems

Michael W. Coates

A veterinary practice management system (PMS) is a specially designed software suite which supports the functioning of the practice and which records electronically virtually all of a practice's service and business activities. PMS functionality includes appointment bookings, stock control, financial processing, invoicing, marketing and case-management features such as X-rays and laboratory test results. PMSs can also be configured to automatically generate client letters, e-mails and reminders, manage reports and facilitate the processing of insurance claims, among other tasks. The primary objective of a PMS is to 'automate' and facilitate the administrative function of a veterinary practice, so that key data are available and accessible quickly and easily: literally, at the touch of a button.

This chapter aims to provide an overview of some key aspects of computer systems management in a veterinary practice. Practice owners and managers need to be aware of their responsibilities in this area, as the computer system is crucial to a practice's effective operation. There are legal requirements that must be met as well.

In the absence of a trained systems administrator, practice managers are often required to carry out basic administrative tasks on the practice network, such as adding and removing users, carrying out regular backups or installing new hardware. The system vendor should provide the necessary training to carry out these basic tasks. For advanced network tasks, however, it is usual to have a contract with the vendor to provide the necessary information technology (IT) support. Everyday administrative tasks are made as easy as possible by software programmers. However, the same user interfaces that are used to accomplish these tasks also allow access to very powerful tools for making large changes to the way that the network operates. As a result, it is essential that only individuals with the necessary knowledge make changes to the servers and user data on a network. It is advisable for managers to seek professional advice in the first instance if they have any doubts about their own abilities to complete specific tasks successfully.

## Security Threats

In these days of sophisticated and interconnected PC networks, together with the increasing value of data as a tradable commodity, security has become a major concern of businesses and home computer users alike. Businesses are required by law to put measures in place to ensure the integrity and security of data, as there are many potential threats to both data and the systems on which the data are stored. 'Data integrity' refers to the data's accuracy, while security concerns control of access to the data.

## Users

Users have the most power to compromise security, sometimes unwittingly. People make mistakes, and this can include accidental deletion or modification of important data. Controlling access to certain data can go some way towards alleviating this problem, but this must be balanced with fair and sensible access to ensure that staff can still perform their jobs. Suitable policies should be developed to allow individuals limited access only to those parts of the system that they need to use in order to do their jobs. Old user accounts, such as ex-employee accounts, can also present a security risk and so these must be disabled, as should any 'guest' computer accounts, because they present an easy method of gaining unauthorized access to the practice's network. Password protocols can increase security. These could include requiring users to change their passwords after a period of time and having complexity requirements, such as requiring passwords to contain a minimum number of characters or specific combinations of characters and numbers.

© C.R. Coates 2012. *Veterinary Practice Management* (C.R. Coates)

## Hardware failure and theft

In general, PCs are very reliable machines, but breakdowns and hardware failure can and do occur. Any maintenance contracts on hardware must be kept up to date, and any contract terms, such as engineer response times in the event of a failure, must be suitable for the practice's needs. Hardware, which may potentially contain important or sensitive data, can also be stolen.

## Accidental damage

Accidental damage to hardware is surprisingly common. Examples include drinks being spilled over equipment and portable devices being dropped. These types of problem are impossible to predict and plan for, and are essentially out of the practice manager's control.

## External factors

Hardware problems can also be caused by external factors, such as fire, floods and lightning – surprisingly common, as computer equipment is sensitive to sudden electrical discharge. Animals, such as mice and squirrels, can chew through cabling.

## Third-party attacks

A practice's computer system, if unsecured, can be used by external individuals to attack other systems. In addition to unprotected data being at risk, it is possible for unscrupulous individuals to utilize a system for sending spam e-mails, launching scams, or even hosting illegal files. System administrators should check systems regularly for signs of external interference. Specialized hardware firewalls and e-mail filters can be purchased to reduce the likelihood of this type of attack.

An example of a third-party attack is the denial-of-service (DoS) attack, which floods target computers or networks with large amounts of unwanted network traffic, thus reducing the network's ability to function normally and causing disruption to users. In a distributed denial-of-service attack (DDoS), third-party networks are hijacked by attackers, who then synchronize many networks to bombard a single target with network traffic. This method also makes it more difficult to identify the location of the attacker. In essence, a third-party attack involves the attacker using the resources of a computer system they do not own for their own illicit purposes.

## Malware

Malware is the term for software that is written for malicious purposes. There are various forms of malware, the most common of which are viruses, Trojans and root kits, all designed to cause malicious damage to a system. In the great majority of cases, malware must have authorization from the computer user before it can enter a system. Because of this, the users of malware often try to disguise malicious software as legitimate e-mail messages. Files attached to e-mail messages are a common method of sending malware programs to unsuspecting users.

## Counteracting Security Threats

There are many forms of software to counter the above threats, which are available from a variety of manufacturers. For most types of software, including software intended for computer security, corporate licences can be obtained that permit the software to be installed on several computers for a one-off fee, as opposed to paying for a licence for each individual computer. This often works out as the most cost-effective procedure, especially for larger practices, where many PCs may be in use.

### Antivirus software

As its name suggests, *antivirus (AV) software* detects and eliminates computer viruses. Modern virus checkers have a number of advanced features, intended to 'catch' viruses at their point of entry into a system, by monitoring Internet links, e-mail attachments and external devices such as USB flash drives. Most virus checkers also include the ability to scan the computer's RAM (random access memory), making it more likely that any virus resident on the system will be detected. In some cases, however, it is not possible for a virus to be completely removed by AV software. In those cases, special 'removal tools' are available from manufacturers of AV software and these will eliminate a particular virus from a system.

### Firewalls

A *firewall* is a piece of software intended to prevent unwanted intrusion into a computer or network.

Intrusion into a system can take the form of a request to read data or otherwise use a system resource, which comes from an unknown computer, normally outside the local network. A firewall can prevent the installation of root kits (see Appendix 1), and also prevent data theft or a system being used for third-party attacks. In larger networks, a computer with two network cards is sometimes configured to be a firewall. This machine normally sits between the Internet and the local network, with all traffic between the local and outside networks going through the machine. Individual PCs also normally have a firewall installed. This may come as part of the operating system, or be provided by a third-party vendor. Many modern AV systems incorporate a firewall, so recently it has become largely unnecessary to purchase separate firewall software.

### Automatic blocking

It is possible to configure most e-mail systems to block attachments with certain file extensions, such as ".exe", which is the most common type of extension found on executable program files. Program files however, must be treated differently from a data file, such as a Word or Excel document. Instead of being opened for viewing or editing, the program code that they contain is executed by the computer's CPU (central processing unit). The default for Windows installations (in more recent versions) is to hide the file extension (and the dot before it) if the file type is known to the operating system. This results in only the first part of the file name being displayed to the user. Any dots elsewhere in the file name will still be displayed however, so a file named <productList.doc.exe> will appear to the user who downloaded the file as <productList.doc>. Using this method, attackers can cause a program to masquerade as a legitimate data file, and when activated the program's action may not be immediately obvious to the user. This often makes it more difficult to trace the source of malicious software on a network. It is possible, however, to configure the operating system not to hide file extensions, which is a wise precaution to prevent the introduction of malicious software to the practice network.

### Software patches

AV software and operating systems should be kept maintained with the latest updates and software 'patches' where necessary. Patches are pieces of software intended to correct a particular issue in a piece of software. They may be also needed to address any hardware incompatibility, but those most commonly required by a veterinary practice (although they also apply to home users) address security issues which are occasionally discovered in databases and operating systems, as well as in other applications used by the practice.

A major reason to keep systems up to date is that many examples of viruses and Trojans exploit software vulnerabilities that have already had patches released to repair the issues. However, in reality, there are enough unprotected home and business computers for viruses to spread. Although not actually part of the practice network, increasing numbers of unprotected computers on the Internet actually increase the likelihood that the practice network will become attacked by malicious software at some point. This may be via the home computers of practice employees, which, if unprotected, could pose a threat to the practice system. For example, a member of staff may plug a removable device, such as a USB flash (pen) drive, into their unprotected home computer, and the pen drive becomes infected; the staff member may then plug the pen drive into a computer on the practice network, thereby infecting the network. Staff training, in conjunction with keeping virus checkers and other software up to date, will reduce the risks of malware being introduced in this manner.

### Staff Training

Despite everyone's best intentions, it is still possible for a system to be compromised if threats are misunderstood. That is why all users of the system should be made aware of the security threats mentioned above. Training users to use the system appropriately and correctly reduces the possibility of problems caused by user error. Thus, all staff should be trained in data security and protection. This training should include the safe use of e-mail and the Internet, as well as password protection. It is advisable to include a written policy for e-mail, Internet and telephone use in the Staff Handbook. An example of such a practice policy can be found in Appendix 2. Staff should also be familiar with the provisions of the Data Protection Act 1998 and with practice protocols for giving clients access to their own and their pets' information. Staff should not be permitted to use CDs or pen drives from unprotected PCs on practice computers, but may use these media if they have been virus checked beforehand. Copying sensitive data and removing it from the premises should be forbidden. Laptops and other mobile devices should not contain any sensitive data at all and should only be able to access the practice database remotely via a password-protected connection.

## Backups

The importance of complete and reliable backups cannot be understated. In addition to providing data security and peace of mind, generating backups is also a legal requirement under the Data Protection Act 1998. While creating backups does not reduce the risks to a system, such backups do allow disaster recovery where data might otherwise be permanently lost. Owing to the large number of hazards, it is inevitable that a practice will face data loss problems at some point, even with the best maintenance and user training. In many cases where equipment has been damaged or has failed, data can be recovered from it. However, specialist equipment is required for this purpose and this type of data recovery can be extremely expensive.

The principle of back ups is to make a copy of important data stored on the system, so that the data may be restored in the event of a disaster. Backups can also be used to restore files that have been accidentally deleted or modified. Many devices can be used to back up data, from flash drives for small amounts of data, to hard disk and tape drives. Tapes are created for the specific purpose of backups and take the form of plastic cartridges with capacities of several hundred gigabytes. They are generally preferred for backups as tape cartridges are far more robust than a hard disk drive, and also easier to store and transport.

The time taken to back up a system will vary hugely between systems. It may take only a few minutes to back up a small system, while it can take several hours to back up a large corporate system. Because of the load on the hard disks being backed up, system performance can be impeded while the backup is running. Because of this, as well as the time taken, backups are normally carried out overnight. Tapes should be changed every day, and it is also advisable to have at least five tapes for a particular backup. This results in far better data security, as a backup may not complete successfully, for example because of hardware error, or the backup tapes themselves can fail. It is recommended that tapes be replaced at the interval set by the manufacturer. When they are not in use, the tapes (or other backup media) should ideally be kept in a safe on the premises or off site.

## Upgrading Computer Systems

In the early years of PCs, it was normal to regularly conduct large-scale hardware upgrades in order to have the ability to run the latest software, which often had extremely useful new features not present in older versions, or which required a specific type of system to make use of these features. All PCs would be replaced as frequently as every 2–3 years. More recently, however, with computers still rapidly increasing in processing power, the features offered by software are limited more by the imagination of the programmers and the constraints of any particular operating system than by the ability of the hardware to process data and perform advanced tasks, as was previously the case. In addition to this, the vast increase in the use of computer networks has caused the practice network to become viewed as a single system, rather than as a collection of individual computers. The prevalence of networks has also resulted in more data processing being conducted by servers, as opposed to individual workstations.

This shift from standalone PCs to networks has turned the process of upgrading systems into more of a gradual evolution. This evolution has also been enhanced by the backward compatibility of PC hardware and software. Due to compatibility between older and new systems, it is possible for a network to originally have been set up to use a particular version of Microsoft Windows, but for newer versions to be installed on top of this. For example, Windows XP was surpassed by Windows Vista, which itself was replaced by Windows 7. Owing to backward compatibility (meaning that newer operating systems can run older software, and applications can read files created by older versions of the program), a new Windows 7-based PC is able to connect to and use the resources of a Windows XP-based network. As a result, it is becoming easier to integrate new systems into the network, with the consequence that a practice may have various operating systems on the same network. However, from the manager's perspective, it is important that all systems have the latest updates for both the operating systems involved and AV software.

For most tasks required by a practice, a 10-year-old PC will still do the job, although newer PCs tend to be faster and easier to operate. PC hardware eventually fails for a variety of reasons. If systems are not kept clean and free of dust inside the case, vents and heat sinks can become clogged, which can lead to the PC overheating, which greatly reduces the lifetime of the components. PCs also contain mechanical components, such as hard disk drives, fans and optical drives. These can fail, leading to loss of data (in the case of a hard disk), or the overheating of components and a potentially broken CPU or motherboard. In larger practices with several large servers, adequate cooling is essential, as these large PCs generate considerable amounts of heat. Generally, hardware failures tend to affect older computers. In these cases, the cost of repair can far exceed the value of the system, and it is less disruptive to the practice and cheaper to replace the machine with a new one.

As a result of the modular construction of PCs, it is reasonably easy to conduct minor upgrades on ageing systems, such as adding more memory or a more modern optical drive, for example, a writable DVD drive to replace a CD-ROM drive. This can increase the operating lifetime of older systems, and is normally cost-effective. Removal of dust from the insides of computers at least once a year can also increase component lifetimes and ensure continued reliability of systems. Note that cleaning electrical components, such as those found in computers, must be done using canned compressed air. Physical contact with components can cause damage, and silicon microchips (which account for many of the components of a PC) can be damaged by static discharge. Walking across a carpet can cause a person to build up a static charge, and this can be released through components, causing significant damage. For this reason, it is advisable to conduct hardware upgrades in a static-free environment, preferably with no carpets, and a good earthed object (for example a radiator or copper pipe). The PC chassis should be attached to ground, and it is also recommended that the individual performing the upgrade uses an earthed wrist strap.

On occasion, a large system upgrade is required, which may include replacing servers with newer systems, or replacing large numbers of PCs. In these cases, it is necessary to plan the upgrade in advance. This involves predicting any possible difficulties that may be encountered during the upgrade, including the migration of user files and data, as well as any compatibility issues. Any work required as part of the upgrade that requires physical access to systems, or a loss of availability resulting from servers being offline, must be timed well for minimal disruption to the practice. This may involve carrying out the upgrading outside the practice's opening hours. Sometimes, it is necessary to run the old and new systems together for a time, while data can be transferred to the new system, and users can be trained in its use. Running the two systems simultaneously also allows the new system to be thoroughly tested before the original system is eventually taken offline. Another advantage of doing this is that problems in moving large amounts of data can be overcome with less disruption to the practice, although it does increase the overall length of time required to complete the upgrade.

## Computers and the Law

As the use of computers has spread, laws have been introduced which define misuse of a system, protect program code from unauthorized use, and ensure that the personal information of individuals is not used incorrectly and is accurate. In the UK, there are several Acts of Parliament that are of importance to any business which holds data electronically and to individuals using computers.

### Copyright, Designs and Patents Act 1988

Copyright law makes it illegal to download or redistribute music, books or software electronically without permission from the copyright holder. Software is protected for up to 50 years after the death of the author. Software licences originated from the desire by software manufacturers to ensure that each copy of their software is only run on one computer and is not copied for the use of others. To ensure that a practice has software with valid licences, a software audit can be carried out. This normally involves using audit software run from a server, which is able to detect software used on networked computers and to assess whether any licences that are required are valid. Software copyright and licensing is significantly less of a concern on systems that utilize open-source software and operating systems, because copyright and licensing does not apply to these systems.

## Computer Misuse Act 1990

This Act mainly concerns data and crimes associated with unauthorized data manipulation, making it an offence to access computer-based data without authorization. Such access includes access in order to commit or facilitate the commission of an offence. Unauthorized modification of data is also illegal, although in order to modify data, an individual must first gain unauthorized access to it.

## Police and Justice Act 2006

This Act includes some important additions to the Computer Misuse Act 1990. Under the 2006 legislation, any act intending to impair the operation of a computer is a criminal offence, carrying a maximum penalty of 10 years. Creating, adapting or supplying 'any article' with the intention, belief or knowledge that it will be used to commit an offence is also illegal. Although not specific to computing, 'any article' can refer to computer programs and data. This could include items on CDs, DVDs or flash drives if they contain malware or illegally copied software, music or films.

## Data Protection Act 1998

This Act of Parliament deals with holding data electronically, and specifically applies to data pertaining to private individuals (clients of the practice, and also staff). The key provisions of the Data Protection Act 1998 can be summarized in the eight key 'principles of data protection', which are as follows:

- Data must only be used for the specific purposes for which it was collected.
- Unless there is legislation or other overriding legitimate reason to share information (for example, the prevention or detection of a crime), data can only be passed to other parties with consent of the individual the data is about. It is an offence for other parties to obtain this personal data without authorization.
- Individuals have a right to access the information held about them, subject to certain exceptions (for example, information held for the prevention or detection of a crime).
- Personal information may not be kept for longer than is necessary and must be kept up to date.

- Personal information may not be sent outside the European Economic Area unless the individual whom it is about has consented or unless adequate protection is in place, for example, by the use of a prescribed form of contract to govern the transmission of the data.
- Other than for very simple processing, and for domestic use, all entities that process personal information must register with the Information Commissioner's Office.
- A company that is holding personal information is required to have adequate security measures in place. Those include technical measures (such as backups) and organizational measures (such as staff training).
- Subjects have the right to have factually incorrect information about them corrected (note: this does not extend to matters of opinion)

## Conclusions

As has been shown, computer systems are subject to a number of serious threats, and it is the practice owner's and manager's responsibility to protect the practice system and data from these. Specific threats include user errors and malicious attacks, hardware failure and theft, third-party attacks and malware. AV software will protect the system from most of these threats, as will appropriate server settings and configuration, as well as staff training in the safe and correct use of the system. The importance of carrying out regular backups of the system and data cannot be overstated. Backups allow recovery of the system and data in the event of a major disaster and should be carried out at the same time every day. Backup media should be stored safely and checked for integrity regularly.

All hardware should be kept free from dust and serviced. From time to time PCs will need to be upgraded. A cost-effective method of doing this is to upgrade components rather than the entire machine. In the case of an entire system upgrade, it is necessary to plan this in advance. Planning involves predicting any possible difficulties that may be encountered during the upgrade, including the migration of user files and data, as well as any compatibility issues.

In the UK, computers and data are subject to a number of legal requirements, which must be complied with, and it is the responsibility of practice owners and managers to ensure this compliance.

## Further Information

See Appendix 1: Computer Terminology Explained.

## Revision Questions

1. Explain the difference between antivirus software and a firewall.
2. Describe the responsibilities of the practice manager in relation to computers and data.
3. What training in data protection and security is provided to staff at your practice? Is this training effective in preventing user-caused problems?
4. Describe two specific computer-related problems that have occurred in your practice, and which you were aware of. Analyse the causes of these problems and the effectiveness of the solutions that were applied. Are you confident that these problems will not reoccur?

# SECTION 4
# Financial Management – A Matter for the Accountant?

### Section Objectives

At the end of this section, you should be able to:

- Explain the factors, both internal and external, that have an impact on practice profitability.
- Explain the different ways in which a business can increase profits.
- Explain the difference between financial and management accounting.
- Analyse basic financial accounts.
- Evaluate a business's performance using key accounting ratios and performance indicators.

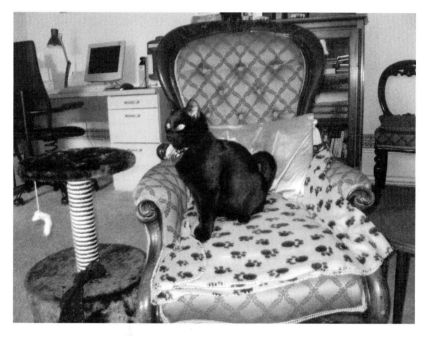

20% of UK households own a cat (PFMA Survey, 2011).

# 16 Profitability

## What is Profit?

Veterinary practices earn income from the services they provide to clients and from sales of drugs, medicines and pet products. In order to earn this income, they must also incur costs. Table 16.1 shows a breakdown of typical sources of income and costs in a small animal veterinary practice (in no particular order).

Veterinary practices do not make their own drugs, medicines, surgical consumables or pet food and so must buy these goods in from suppliers. These goods are listed both as a cost and as a source of income, because the majority are bought for resale and so the cost is recouped from sales. Drugs and medicines costs are classed as direct costs of sales.

In order for a practice to survive, the income it earns must cover all of its costs. The sum remaining after all of the costs have been paid must be sufficient to enable the owner/s to pay taxes owing, repay loans and put by funds for replacement equipment, as well as leaving a suitable sum for themselves, as a return for the investment they made when setting up the business.

Thus, profit is the sum left over from income after all business expenses have been paid. It is an absolute value, calculated by deducting a practice's costs from its income. Businesses calculate their profit regularly throughout the financial year – usually on a monthly basis – and at the end of a financial year they calculate the profit for the entire year.

Profitability concerns the longer term prospects of a business and its ability to generate profits consistently year on year. It is a relative measure – a practice will assess its own performance by looking at the changes to the rate of return on investment, and the gross and net profit margins, over time. It will also make comparisons with its direct competitors and available industry statistics, which are used as a benchmark to gauge how well it is performing compared with the rest of the industry. It is essential that a business maintains its capacity to earn a profit year on year, but there are many factors, both internal and external, which determine both the level of profit and a business's capacity to generate profit consistently.

## Factors Affecting Profitability

The level of profit which a practice can potentially earn is determined by a range of factors:

- The type and location of the practice
- The level of competition the practice faces
- The prices clients are willing and able to pay
- The business skills and aptitude and ambition of the owners
- The profitability of the industry sector as a whole

### Type of practice

Small animal practices are the most numerous in the UK, representing approximately 54% of all practices (RCVS, 2011). Mixed practices are the next largest category (12%), followed by large animal (4%) and equine practices (3%), although these percentages are not exact. Turnover per full-time equivalent veterinarian tends to be higher in small animal practice than in mixed practice. Mixed practices also have a greater reliance on sales of drugs and medicines as a source of income than do small animal practices (British Veterinary Association, 2003).

In small animal practice, clients generally bring their animals to the practice and the veterinarian can see a large number of pets in a day. However, the average individual transaction value is relatively small and so this must be offset by larger numbers of pets seen. The relative costs of providing services are correspondingly lower. In contrast, large animal and equine practice veterinarians

**Table 16.1.** Sources of small animal veterinary practice income and costs.

| Income | Costs |
|---|---|
| • Consultations | • Salaries and wages |
| • Operations | • Drugs, medicines and |
| • Dental treatments | pet products |
| • Procedures (e.g. lumps, wounds, anal glands, vaccinations, etc.) | • Power – i.e. electricity, gas (for heating and lighting and to operate equipment) |
| • Sales of drugs, medicines, pet products | • Water |
| • Sales of pet foods | • Council tax |
| • Nurse clinics | • Laboratory costs |
| • Behaviour classes | • Repairs and maintenance |
| • Other | • Computing |
| | • Telephones |
| | • Advertising |
| | • Bank charges |
| | • Cleaning |
| | • Insurances |
| | • Vehicles |
| | • Health and safety (including radiation and anaesthetic gas exposure monitoring) |
| | • Administration |
| | • Recruitment costs |
| | • Postage |
| | • Staff training |
| | • Other |

spend most of their time seeing animals on clients' premises, so the time taken up in travelling to and treating animals *in situ* means that a relatively small number of visits can be made in a day. Average transaction values are higher, however, because there are more animals and large animal and equine veterinarians must recover their travel costs as well as the costs of any veterinary treatment and drugs provided.

Most dog and cat owners acquire their pets for companionship (PFMA, 2008) and new pets quickly become members of the family. Because of this special bond, cat and dog owners are willing to spend greater amounts of money on their pets and are more likely to consent to expensive or complex treatment in order to prolong their pets' lives, so income for small animal practices is easier to earn. Also, small animal practice clients are accustomed to paying at the time of treatment, so cash flow is more easily managed. In contrast, farm animals are a commodity and farmers have

to contend with a large number of external pressures and legislative requirements in order to breed and keep these animals. They are more reluctant to call the veterinarian out and are less likely to incur large veterinary fees unless this is absolutely necessary. Farms are businesses and so they expect to be invoiced for services rendered and expect reasonable credit terms. Thus, for large animal veterinarians, earning a profit and managing client debt is a greater challenge. For equine veterinarians, the scenario is similar. Although horse owners tend to be better off financially because owning horses is expensive, they are generally reluctant to pay higher fees if the horse is not a valuable animal. In addition, a much smaller percentage of UK households owns a horse compared with households that own dogs and cats, so limiting the potential for increasing profits in equine practice.

## Location of practice

Simmons (1997) argues that location is crucial to practice success and this is becoming more so as time progresses. There are two key influences – geographical location and client demographics. According to Simmons, practice growth is dependent on residential growth. Therefore, a practice located in a high-growth area will also experience growth, as client numbers continue to increase. However, in the longer term, this growth will eventually slow or halt so profits in that longer term may not be assured. Well-established practices operating in mature areas, where there is little growth, may have built up considerable goodwill and a satisfactory compliment of loyal clients over time, but will have limited growth potential in the longer term.

Urban practices may need to cover a much larger area than rural practices, because dog and cat ownership in urban areas is lower. Urban practices may also suffer increased client turnover and higher running costs than rural practices.

The demographic characteristics that influence practice profits are the number of households, household composition and age, annual income and type of housing. Pet numbers will depend on the number of households present within the area served by the practice (generally within a 5–10 mile radius). In the UK, one in two households owns a pet, so the more households a practice serves, the more pets there are to treat.

In 2007, Murray *et al.* (2010) carried out a study that investigated the number and ownership profiles of cats and dogs in the UK. Among other findings, their results showed that households with gardens were more likely to own cats and dogs than households without gardens. They also found that dog ownership increased as household size increased and that dogs were more likely to be owned by rural households. A strong relationship was discovered between dog ownership and households that included children aged between 11 and 15 years. Families with five or more occupants and families with children over the age of five were more likely to own a dog than households with fewer occupants or with very young children. Cats were more likely to be owned by households living in semi-urban or rural areas.

## Client spending

Simmons (1997) also observes that the likelihood of a pet owner incurring veterinary fees varies directly with household income. Disposable income determines the level of discretionary spending on pets and so the higher the income, the higher the level of discretionary spending. However, a very high income area is likely to be less populated and so although the average transaction fee might be higher, there will be fewer transactions than in a middle-income area with a higher household count. Simmons cites his own experience of middle-income neighbourhoods, in which 65% to 75% of pet owners will incur annual veterinary fees. Therefore, middle-income neighbourhoods are likely to generate the greatest proportion of a practice's income.

## Level of competition

Neighbouring practices which treat the same species pose the greatest threat, so a practice that is obliged to share the same client base with another will find it harder to make a profit and will have to maintain a consistent effort to keep its existing clients.

Over the past 10 years, the UK has seen the rise of joint-venture partnerships and corporate practices. These organizations can achieve economies of scale by centralizing purchasing, human resources, and administrative and accounting functions. Veterinarians are employed by them, but are also offered profit sharing as an incentive to grow the practices they manage. For the individual veterinarian who is put off by the responsibility and complexity of running his/her own business, the option of becoming one's own boss, but without the risk, is very attractive.

Pet superstores, operating both in large premises and online, can stock and sell a huge variety of pet products at cheaper prices, once again benefiting from economies of scale and greater purchasing power. Supermarkets and wholesalers have sold pet foods and pet products for a very long time now, and continue to compete with veterinary practices, both on price and variety. Online pharmacies sell veterinary drugs and medicines more cheaply and owners of pets on long-term medication, in particular, are switching to such suppliers.

Thus, clients have a much greater choice when it comes to pet products and pet foods and from whom they buy their drugs and medicines. Hence, practices need to look to the veterinary services they provide, and the things that only veterinarians are qualified and licensed to do, as the main source of their income, rather than relying on sales of drugs and products.

## Business skills, aptitude and ambition of owners

Two neighbouring practices with similar veterinary expertise and facilities, competing for the same client base, can earn different levels of income such that one ends up being more profitable than the other. The reason for this difference more often than not lies in the comparative skills, aptitudes and ambitions of the practice owners themselves. To run a successful practice requires a great deal of knowledge, to which this text and others attest. Much of the necessary skills and knowledge can be gained on the job through experience, but a considerable amount, particularly marketing, finance and leadership, requires the owner to put in the necessary effort to learn. Effective owners will understand this and will make that effort. Others, though, will fail to appreciate the need, with the inevitable consequences.

An owner who is not content with simply maintaining the status quo, but wants the practice to grow and evolve, will seek ways to achieve this. Such owners will be more open to innovative approaches and will not be afraid of change. They will also seek ways to improve processes and the veterinary service they provide – anticipating client needs rather than simply responding to them.

### Profitability of the industry

Porter (2008) argues that the profitability of an industry results from the interaction of five key competitive forces – existing competitors, the bargaining power of suppliers, the bargaining power of buyers, the threat of substitute products and the threat of new entrants. According to Porter, the rivalry that results from these five forces shapes the structure of the industry and determines its profitability (Fig. 16.1). Porter argues that these five forces are the key drivers of profitability within an industry and in order to understand profitability within one's own industry, one must carry out an analysis of these forces. Some forces may not be as powerful as others, but if collectively they are powerful, then most businesses within the industry will struggle to achieve a good level of return.

### Existing competitors

Veterinary practices in the UK face competition not only from competing practices that treat the same species, but also from supermarkets, wholesalers, pet stores with an in-house veterinarian, online stores and pharmacies. Apart from direct competitors, most of the competition centres around drugs, prophylactic treatments (flea and worming treatments), pet food, other pet products and toys. Competition for the supply of such items is intense.

It makes little sense, therefore, for practices to try to compete with much bigger and more powerful competitors for a share of the pet product and pet food market. Instead, veterinarians are well placed to compete on the basis of clinical veterinary service provision, which only they are qualified and licensed to provide. It is the quality of service provision or the unique way in which it is delivered that will differentiate a veterinary practice from its competitors.

### New entrants to the industry

Over the last 5 years, the UK has witnessed the arrival of joint-venture partnerships, franchises and corporate practices, and an increase in large group practices. The threat to the one-person or small independent or partnership practice from these larger entities is high. Indeed, it could be argued that over the next 5 to 10 years, single-owner veterinary practices and small partnership practices may well cease to exist in the UK. The arrival of these larger business entities has the effect of reducing prices. The corporates can achieve economies of scale and, therefore, can charge less for the services they provide, thus forcing the more traditional practices to try to compete on price. The barriers to entry are high for individuals, because of the considerable capital investment required to open a new practice or even buy an existing one, but these barriers are easily overcome if one joins a joint-venture partnership or buys a franchise, because the initial capital investment required is smaller.

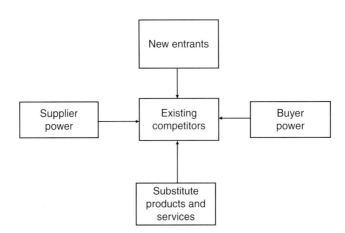

**Fig. 16.1.** Porter's five competitive forces, which define an industry's structure (Porter, 2008).

## Threat of substitute products or services

The Internet is increasingly replacing the veterinarian for owners seeking information and advice about their pet's condition. This means that owners are visiting practices less frequently or are turning instead to alternative therapies, such as herbalism, homeopathy and acupuncture. Farmers have always provided basic veterinary care for their animals and will continue to do so, only calling the veterinarian out for things they cannot handle themselves or when drugs are required that only a veterinarian can prescribe. It is likely that the current economic climate will lead to an increase in this trend as farmers' incomes continue to fall.

## Supplier power

A veterinary practice uses a wide range of suppliers, but two key groups of suppliers are the drugs, medicines and medical consumables suppliers, and the pet food manufacturers, which also supply prescription diets. In the UK, Safavet UK is the market leader supplying the veterinary profession by market share, closely followed by the Dechra Pharmaceuticals group, to which National Veterinary Services and Dechra Veterinary Products, among others, belong. The Dechra group does not rely exclusively on the veterinary industry for its business as it also supplies the human medicines market in the UK and exports to other countries as well. Nevertheless, the veterinary sector represents a significant percentage of its business.

Suppliers have long recognized the importance of the veterinary sector and many work to develop partnerships with practices through providing ancillary services, such as business advice, record keeping and management reporting, all of which have the effect of tying the customer to them. Purchasing from drugs and consumables wholesalers is done electronically and online nowadays, through the use of hand-held devices used in practices alongside barcoding systems, which automate and streamline the ordering process. Once a practice has been locked into a particular supplier's system, though, transferring to another supplier is rather inconvenient. So these large suppliers, relatively few in number, are very powerful because competition is limited. As a result, prices for veterinary drugs and medicines remain high.

Prescription diets can only be prescribed by a veterinarian and so key suppliers of such diets work hard to develop close relationships with veterinarians, starting with undergraduates at veterinary school, in order to build positive associations. Thus, they will provide support to veterinary schools in the form of lectures and sponsorship, and to veterinary practices in the form of business and marketing advice, as well as sponsorship, all of which serve to build positive associations and a 'relationship' that suppliers hope will last in the longer term.

## Client power

Clients are powerful, because without clients a practice could not exist. Also, clients can easily transfer to another practice if they wish. But once a practice has developed a relationship with the client and their pet, clients are much more reluctant to change. Practices must, therefore, work hard to keep their clients. Most of a practice's marketing efforts are geared towards retaining existing clients rather than towards gaining new clients. Most new clients are gained through word-of-mouth recommendation, so a satisfied client base is the most effective marketing tool (see Section 1).

In conclusion, profit and profitability in veterinary practice are dependent on a wide range of different factors, some of which are within the control of the practice owner, while others are not. The level of profit which a practice can potentially earn is dependent on the characteristics of the client base, the location of the practice, the nature of direct competition, the skills and abilities and ambition of the practice owner and the profitability of the veterinary industry as a whole. The structure of the veterinary industry determines the industry's overall profitability. The key factors that drive an industry's profitability are the nature of the rivalry between direct competitors, the power of suppliers and clients, the threat of new entrants and the threat of substitute products. An understanding of the industry and of the influence of these competing factors enables better informed strategic decision making by managers.

## References

British Veterinary Association (2003) Trends in practice performance, 2000–2002. In Practice 25, 556–558.

Murray, J.K., Browne, W.J., Roberts, M.A., Whitmarsh, A. and Gruffydd-Jones, T.J. (2010) Number and ownership profiles of cats and dogs in the UK. Veterinary Record 166, 163–168.

PFMA (2008) Pet Ownership Trends 2011. Pet Food Manufacturers' Association, London. Available at http://www.pfma.org.uk/pet-ownership-trends/ (accessed 13 March 2012).

Porter, M.E. (2008) The five competitive forces that shape strategy. *Harvard Business Review* 86(1), January 2008, 78–93.

RCVS (2011) *RCVS Facts 2011, The Annual Report of The Royal College of Veterinary Surgeons: Part 2.* Royal College of Veterinary Surgeons, London. Available at: http://www.rcvs.org.uk/publications/rcvs-facts-2011/rcvsfacts2011.pdf (accessed 30 May 2012).

Simmons, J.L. (1997) *Veterinary Practice Management – Building Profit and Value.* Mosby-Year Book, St Louis, Missouri.

## Revision Questions

**1.** With reference to a veterinary practice with which you are familiar, carry out an analysis of the internal and external factors that influence the practice's profitability.

**2.** Select four key practice stakeholders and assess their relative power and influence on practice profitability. Which, in your opinion, is the most important stakeholder? Justify your view.

**3.** Select five suppliers from whom the practice buys goods and products (excluding food). Evaluate the relationship between the practice and these suppliers and identify the ways in which they attempt to tie the practice to them.

**4.** Review the types of pet food that the practice sells and establish the rationale behind the choice of stock. If your practice sells only one brand of food, establish the nature of the practice's relationship with the supplier and identify the specific ways in which the practice benefits from this relationship.

**5.** If you were to consider setting up your own practice today, what would be the barriers that would prevent you from doing so and how might these be overcome?

# 17 The Profit and Loss Account

Every business owner and manager should have a good understanding of two key financial statements which are prepared by businesses at the end of every financial year in accordance with the accounting regulations and protocols in operation in the country within which the business trades. These two statements are the 'Profit and Loss Account' (also known as the 'Trading and Profit and Loss Account') and the 'Balance Sheet'. The balance sheet will be discussed in detail in the next chapter (Chapter 18).

## What is a Profit and Loss Account?

An example of a profit and loss (P&L) account is given in Table 17.1.

The P&L account is a financial summary of the trading activities of a business for the preceding 12 month period – the income earned and the expenditure incurred during that period, detailed by income and expenditure type. The financial year of a business begins and ends on the same dates each year; the start date is set when the business first started trading and the end date is 12 calendar months from the start date. Thus, a business whose financial year began on the 1 June 2011 will have a year-end date of 31 May 2012.

## Where do the Figures for the P&L Account Come From?

Financial record-keeping systems are run on the dual-entry principle, which means that every transaction is entered twice, in two different accounts. For example, if a practice bought some drugs on credit from a drug wholesaler for resale to clients, this purchase would be entered in the Purchases account (as a debit) to show that drugs have been received into stock, and again in the wholesaler's account (as a credit) to show that the wholesaler is

owed payment for them; or if an administrator bought a pack of envelopes for a mailing and paid for these in cash, the transaction would be entered into the Stationery account (as a debit) to show that stationery had been received and, again, in the Petty Cash book (as a credit) to show that petty cash had been spent.

At the end of a financial period, the balances of all of the accounts are calculated and a list of accounts and their balances, called a Trial Balance, is produced. If the total of all the debit balances equals the total of all the credit balances, the double entries have been made correctly. This does not mean, however, that no errors have been made at all, because some errors cannot be revealed by this system, such as, for example, making the correct entries in the wrong accounts or entering (correctly) the wrong amount.

The figures from the trial balance are used to produce the P&L account and the balance sheet, but first some of the figures have to be adjusted to ensure that the amounts pertaining to the year that is being reported are correct. For example, if insurance has been paid for a period extending beyond the year-end date, the amount that has been 'overpaid' or prepaid has to be deducted in order to show the correct insurance figure for the year; or if repairs have been carried out, but have not yet been paid for, the repairs figure has to be increased by the amount owing in order to obtain the correct figure for repairs for the year.

## What Does the P&L Account Show?

The P&L account shows the gross profit and the net profit earned for the year. Businesses compare the year's profit with those of previous years in order to establish whether profits are increasing or falling. If the latter, the reasons will be investigated so that steps can be taken to prevent this happening in future years, if possible. It must be noted that the

**Table 17.1.** X and Y Veterinary Practice: Profit and Loss (P&L) Account for the year ended 31 May 2012.

| | £ | £ | £ |
|---|---|---|---|
| Sales (or turnover) | | 845,000 | |
| **Less cost of sales:** | | | |
| Opening stock | 35,000 | | |
| Purchases | 203,000 | | |
| Internal laboratory costs | 22,000 | | |
| External laboratory fees | 32,000 | | |
| Closing stock | (38,000) | (254,000) | |
| **Gross profit** | | | **591,000** |
| **Less expenses:** | | | |
| Salaries and wages | 267,250 | | |
| Vehicle costs | 32,000 | | |
| Council tax | 9,500 | | |
| Insurances | 4,500 | | |
| Light and heat | 6,800 | | |
| Repairs | 25,000 | | |
| Disposals and cremations | 7,723 | | |
| Stationery and postage | 3,365 | | |
| Advertising/marketing costs | 5,500 | | |
| Telephone and Internet | 9,895 | | |
| Staff training | 7,220 | | |
| Bank charges | 10,550 | | |
| Bad debts | 3,250 | | |
| Legal and professional fees | 4,250 | | |
| Depreciation | 12,376 | | |
| Clinical waste disposal | 6,500 | | |
| Cleaning | 6,220 | | |
| Subscriptions | 935 | (422,834) | |
| **Net profit** | | **168,166** | |

P&L account is a historical account based on past activity, so nothing can be done to improve a poor profit already made. That is why it is essential that business owners monitor financial performance throughout the year rather than waiting until the end of the year when the final accounts are produced. Many businesses produce a P&L account on a monthly basis for monitoring purposes, and modern computerized accounting packages make this a relatively straightforward task.

Let us examine the components of the P&L account in more detail.

### Gross profit

Accountants define gross profit as follows:

Gross profit = Sales – Cost of sales

Alternative terms for 'Sales' are 'Turnover' or 'Income'. Small animal veterinary practice income mainly consists of veterinary fees earned and income from the sales of drugs, medicines, food and pet products. Any refunds to clients made during the year (referred to in accounting as 'sales returns') need to be deducted from the sales figure to give the true figure for the year. The cost of sales figure is obtained by adding up all the direct variable costs that are clearly attributable to sales. For example, internal and external laboratory costs are incurred directly as part of the veterinary service provided. Drugs and medicines can only be sold if a practice first buys them in, so these purchases are also included in the 'cost of sales' figure. However, there is always a stock of drugs and medicines left over from the previous year, which will be sold during the next year. This 'opening stock' figure is, therefore, added to the purchases figure and then any stock remaining at the end of the year is deducted to give the true cost of drugs sales made during the current year.

A very high gross profit percentage coupled with a low net profit percentage suggests that this practice's expenses are high and probably need investigating. A quick glance at the practice's expenses reveals that salaries represent around 63% of the total practice expenses, which is very high. Generally, for a small animal practice, a net profit of around 25% may be more acceptable, so this practice should be looking to reduce its costs in order to increase its net profit percentage.

To summarize, the P&L account shows the gross and net profit for a business for a specified period of time, usually one financial year. Gross profit is calculated by deducting the cost of sales from the sales (or turnover) figure. Net profit is calculated by deducting practice expenses from the gross profit figure. A practice can increase its profits by increasing sales, reducing expenses or applying a combination of both measures. The gross profit percentage and the net profit percentage are measures of the profitability of a business. A high gross profit percentage coupled with a low net profit percentage indicates that practice expenses are too high, and that the causes of this may need investigating. Practices calculate their gross profit percentages differently and so it is important to know the basis for the calculation made before making comparisons between similar practices.

## References

Ackerman, L. (2003) *Management Basics for Veterinarians*. ASJA Press, Lincoln, Nebraska.

Shilcock, M. and Stutchfield, G. (2008) *Veterinary Practice Management: A Practical Guide*, 2nd edn. Saunders Elsevier, Edinburgh, UK.

Volk, J.O., Felsted, K.E., Cummings, R.F., Slocum, J.W., Cron, W.L., Ryan, K.G. and Moosbrugger, M.C. (2005) Executive summary of the AVMA–Pfizer business practices study. *Journal of the American Veterinary Medicine Association* 226, 212–218.

## Revision Questions

**1.** ABC Veterinary Practice reported sales worth £165,000 for the year ended 31 July 2012. However, sales returns were £25,000 and practice expenses totalled £105,000. The cost of sales figure was £15,000. Calculate the gross and net profits for this practice. (*To check your answer, refer to Appendix 3.*)

**2.** In a practice with which you are familiar, what recent measures were taken to improve revenues? Explain the specific strategies applied and whether these were (or are) being effective in improving practice performance.

**3.** Find out how the latest price increases were implemented in your foster practice, by whom and when. Talk to the receptionists and find out if there was any significant client reaction to the increases.

**4.** ABC Veterinary Practice decided to sell more wormers and flea products this year, but to keep the prices the same as last year, despite a price rise of 2% imposed by their supplier and additional costs incurred in marketing the products. Speculate as to the likely effect of this strategy on the final profit obtained from the sale of these products.

# 18 The Balance Sheet

Wood and Sangster (1999) describe the 'Balance Sheet' as a list of assets, liabilities and capital, which together represent the financial position of a business on a particular date. Ackerman (2002) and Shilcock and Stutchfield (2008) describe it as a 'snapshot' of a practice's finances on a particular date, usually the last day of the financial year of a business.

At any one time, a veterinary practice will owe money to its suppliers (known as creditors) and will have money owed to it by some of its clients (known as debtors). It may also owe money to the tax authorities and others. The practice owns equipment, vehicles, computers and furniture, and may also own the premises within which it operates. It utilizes these things in the course of its day-to-day activities. Amounts owing by a business to other parties are broadly classed as 'liabilities'. Items and amounts owned by a business, whether equipment or cash in the bank, are classed as 'assets'. When a business is closed, the assets are used to pay off or clear the liabilities. The amount remaining after this is done is repaid to the owner of the business and is called 'capital'. Therefore, capital is the difference between the assets of a business and its liabilities and represents the value of the owner's investment. The owners' capital is increased by the annual profits that a business makes, which are added to the capital on the balance sheet. Likewise, the owner's capital is reduced by withdrawals of money ('drawings') by the owner from the business for his or her own use during the year. At least that is how it looks on paper! In reality, it can happen that when a business is closed, its assets may not be worth very much at all, such that there are insufficient funds to cover the liabilities and the owner walks away at best with nothing or, at worst, liable for the debts of the business.

All of the information concerning a business's assets, liabilities and capital is summarized in a financial statement: the balance sheet. An example of a simplified balance sheet for the two partners X and Y is given in Fig. 18.1. Let us examine the different components of this balance sheet.

## Fixed Assets

A balance sheet usually starts by listing all of the business's fixed assets and the amounts by which they have been depreciated over time. A fixed asset is defined by Wood and Sangster (1999) as an asset that lasts a number of years, that is used by the business in its day-to-day activities and which is not intended for resale. In the balance sheet, fixed assets are usually listed starting with the highest value fixed assets, such as buildings and land, and ending with the fixed assets of lowest value.

Every business should maintain an 'asset register'. This is an up-to-date record of all the fixed assets owned by the business, so it is important to carry out regular audits of practice assets to ensure that the list is current. An individual asset record should contain the following information:

- Date of purchase
- Cost price exclusive of VAT
- The name and address of the supplier
- Details of any current maintenance contracts and of the company providing maintenance support
- The method of depreciation applied and annual depreciation amounts
- Specific consumables required to use the asset, their cost and current supplier
- Asset replacement date (as applicable).

Such a register is essential for planning and capital budgeting purposes and is a fundamental part of good asset management.

Fixed assets are listed in the balance sheet at cost price, i.e. at the price originally paid for the asset. Obviously, over time, an asset's value will change.

© C.R. Coates 2012. *Veterinary Practice Management* (C.R. Coates)

| | £ | £ | £ |
|---|---|---|---|
| | Cost (fixed assets) | Depreciation (fixed assets) | |
| **Fixed assets:** | | | |
| Buildings | 275,000 | 55,000 | 220,000 |
| Fixtures and fittings | 25,000 | 7,500 | 17,500 |
| Surgery equipment | 65,000 | 19,500 | 45,500 |
| Vehicles | 30,000 | 7,500 | 22,500 |
| Computer equipment | 7,500 | 2,475 | 5,025 |
| | 402,500 | 91,975 | 310,525 |
| **Current assets:** | | | |
| Stock of drugs and medicines | | 38,000 | |
| Debtors | 13,723 | | |
| *Less* Provision for bad debts | 1,375 | 12,348 | |
| Bank | | 55,000 | |
| Cash in hand | | 1,500 | |
| Prepayments | | 725 | |
| | | 107,573 | |
| *Less* **Current liabilities:** | | | |
| Creditors | 12,500 | | |
| Accruals | 2,100 | 14,600 | |
| Working capital | | | 92,973 |
| Total assets less current liabilities | | | **403,498** |
| | | | |
| *Financed by:* | | | |
| Long-term liabilities: | | | |
| Bank loan | | | 100,000 |
| Capitals | **Partner X** | **Partner Y** | |
| | 100,000 | 100,000 | 200,000 |
| Current Accounts | | | |
| Balance 1 June 2011 | 45,000 | 55,000 | |
| *Add* Salary | 7,000 | 7,000 | |
| *Add* Share of profit (from P&L account) | 52,083 | 52,083 | |
| | 104,083 | 114,083 | |
| *Less* Drawings | 50,793 | 63,875 | |
| | | | |
| | 53,290 | 50,208 | 103,498 |
| | | | **403,498** |

**Fig. 18.1.** X and Y Veterinary Practice: Balance Sheet as at 31 May 2012.

Most fixed assets will lose value (depreciate), but some, such as land and buildings, may fluctuate in value. From an accounting perspective, these fluctuations are ignored while the business is operating, but when it is sold as a going concern, transferred to new owners or closed, the assets have to be revalued in order to establish how much they are actually worth at that point.

## Depreciation of Fixed Assets

The calculation of depreciation of a fixed asset is dependent on the type of asset and how quickly it loses value over time. Some assets, such as cars and computers, depreciate very quickly and so the rate of depreciation that is applied to these will be higher than the rate applied to assets that depreciate more slowly, such as fixtures and fittings and buildings. Beaney and Green (2005) list the following typical rates of depreciation:

| Fixtures and fittings | 10% of cost p.a. |
| Surgery equipment | 15% of cost p.a. |
| Motor vehicles | 25% of cost p.a. |
| Computer equipment | 15% of cost p.a. (others recommend 33%) |

Buildings are also depreciated, irrespective of the fact that they can appreciate in value, and a typical rate of depreciation that is applied to buildings is 4% per annum to represent the maintenance, repairs and upkeep costs incurred.

Depreciation is treated as an expense and so reduces the net profit that a business earns. However, for tax purposes, because depreciation does not represent an actual outlay of cash by the business during the year, it is added back to the net profit figure before the tax owing by the business is calculated.

There are various methods of calculating depreciation, but once a method has been selected, it is important that this is applied consistently each year. The two best known methods are the *straight line method* and the *reducing balance method*.

### The straight line method

Using this method, the useful life of an asset and any residual value it may have at the end of its life are estimated and the asset is written off over the number of years of its useful life by the same amount each year. For example, a motor vehicle originally cost £15,000 to buy. It is estimated that the vehicle would last for 6 years before needing to be replaced and that at the end of that time, it would have a minimal residual value of approximately £600. Using the straight line method, depreciation is calculated as follows:

£15,000 *less* £600 residual value = £14,400

£14,400 must be written off over a period of 6 years, therefore:

£14,400 ÷ 6 = £2400 must be deducted from the cost of the asset each year for the next 6 years.

### The reducing balance method

Using this method, a fixed percentage is deducted from the reduced cost of the asset each year until the estimated residual value is reached. The formula

used to calculate this percentage is as follows (Wood and Sangster, 1999):

Rate of depreciation $(r) = 1 - \sqrt[n]{s \div c}$

where $n$ represents the number of years over which the depreciation occurs, $s$ the residual value and $c$ the cost of the asset. So, for the motor vehicle above:

$r = 1 - \sqrt[6]{600 \div £15,000} = 1 - 0.584 = 0.415$
$= 42\%$ (rounding up)

Thus, the calculation of depreciation for each of the 6 years of use of the vehicle will be:

| Cost of vehicle | | £15,000 |
|---|---|---|
| Year 1 depreciation | 42% of £15,000 | £6,300 |
| | Balance of cost still to be apportioned | £8,700 |
| Year 2 depreciation | 42% of £8,700 | £3,654 |
| | Balance of cost still to be apportioned | £5,046 |
| Year 3 depreciation | 42% of £5,046 | £2,119 |
| | Balance of cost still to be apportioned | £2,927 |
| Year 4 depreciation | 42% of £2,927 | £1,229 |
| | Balance of cost still to be apportioned | £1,698 |
| Year 5 depreciation | 42% of £1,698 | £713 |
| | Balance of cost still to be apportioned | £985 |
| Year 6 depreciation | 42% of £985 | £414 |
| | Residual value (approximate) | £571 |

While the straight line method deducts a fixed amount for depreciation from the cost of the asset each year, the reducing balance method deducts a higher amount at the start and a smaller amount in later years. It is argued that this method represents a more accurate picture of the use of the asset over time, as when an asset is new, there are few maintenance and repair costs, but as it ages, these costs increase and so are balanced out by reducing depreciation charges (Wood and Sangster, 1999).

### Current Assets

Current assets are cash in hand and at the bank, debtors who are expected to clear their debts within a year, and stock that is expected to be sold during the year. Any expenses that have been prepaid

# 19 Accounting Ratios and Financial Performance Indicators

An important responsibility of any business owner and manager is interpreting, understanding and acting upon financial data. An accountant or business adviser can give advice, but it would be a mistake to rely solely on the judgement of these professionals, the main reason being that no-one can know the practice as well as those who live and work in it every day and who may have done so over a number of years.

Every business, no matter how small, is a complex mix of interrelated processes and activities, transactions, actions and reactions. The figures generated by the accounting system include only those activities that can be expressed in monetary terms. What is more, figures can be manipulated, interpreted and reinterpreted to show different things and, from time to time, they can simply be incorrect. It is imperative, therefore, for those who make the decisions to possess a sound understanding and knowledge of financial information. At the very least, they should know what questions to ask about how the data is generated, where it comes from and what it means.

Financial business data should always be interpreted with reference to the context within which the business operates – the overall profitability of the industry sector as a whole, the external environmental factors that have an impact upon the business, both in the immediate and the wider environments, and industry norms. Comparisons with similar types of practice, if data can be obtained, are also very useful. Benchmarking data are available that show what is happening within the different sectors of the veterinary industry throughout the UK; these can serve the purposes of comparison as well, but such data should not dictate a practice's future performance targets or the methods by which the practice should earn its income, because every individual practice has its own unique set of circumstances, not the least of which is the owner's view of and approach to profit.

## Analysing Financial Accounts

The information contained in the 'Profit and Loss Account' and the 'Balance Sheet' can be analysed in a number of different ways to provide deeper insights into how the business is performing.

Naturally, the current year's accounts will be compared with last year's, and those of the year before that, going as far back as desired. Line-by-line comparisons can be made between the different items, noting the changes over time. Decisions are made depending on the results of these comparisons. If practice income continues to increase year on year, this is obviously a positive trend and one which, it is hoped, the practice owners can clearly link to the decisions they make. If expenses also continue to increase, but by a reasonable amount, which appears to be in line with inflation, this is also positive. This kind of analysis is known as 'horizontal analysis'.

'Trend analysis' takes horizontal analysis a step further and gives the first set of accounts in the series that is being examined a weighting of 100 and then relates all subsequent sets to the base of 100. This enables changes to be seen much more easily than when comparing the actual amounts (Dyson, 1994).

Another method of analysis is called 'vertical analysis' and involves taking each of the profit and loss and balance sheet items and expressing them as a percentage of the totals to which they contribute. For example, if debtors in a balance sheet total £35,000 and the total of current assets is £70,000, then debtors would comprise 50% of the total current assets; this provides a 'relational' basis for comparisons.

'Ratio analysis' is another method of analysis that looks at the relationships between items and expresses that relationship either as a ratio or as a percentage (both are still referred to as 'ratios'). For example, if a practice were to pay off all of its short-term liabilities, it would do so by utilizing its current assets. So, the current asset total is divided by the short-term liabilities total to find what is known as the 'current ratio'. If the ratio of current assets to short-term liabilities is 1:1, then that is a reasonable result. Some argue that, ideally, this ratio should be at least 2:1, but probably no higher. However, this is a debatable point.

Let us look at ratio analysis in more detail.

## Ratio Analysis

Wood and Sangster (2002) argue that ratios make financial information understandable and meaningful to business owners and are a 'first step' towards assessing a business's financial performance because they help to pinpoint items that need further investigation. In ratio analysis, the relationships between key items in the accounts are examined and a simple calculation is performed to express that relationship – usually this is a case of calculating percentages. The key is to ensure that only meaningful relationships are examined. For example, it makes sense to assess the level of debtors in relation to total income earned and then to express debtors as a percentage of income, or to assess the efficiency of business operations in terms of how long stocks of drugs and medicines sit on the shelves before being sold, or how many days it takes on average for the practice to obtain payment of an outstanding client debt. Another important point is that ratios are meaningless when looked at in isolation. The business should be analysed by looking at the set of ratios together, as only together can they build a complete picture of business performance.

It is possible to generate a large number of ratios for any business, but that would be a waste of time and would not yield any more meaningful information than the few key ratios that are commonly used in accounting and which are calculated in the same way for all businesses across many different sectors.

There are four main groups of ratios – *profitability*, *liquidity*, *efficiency* and *investment*. Profitability ratios were explained in Chapter 17. The remaining three groups will be explained here.

### Liquidity ratios

Liquidity ratios set out to establish how quickly a business's current assets can be turned into cash. The current ratio is calculated, as already explained, by dividing current assets by current (short-term) liabilities. This ratio is usually expressed as a factor.

Thus, for X and Y Veterinary Practice (see Fig. 18.1), the current ratio is 7:1, indicating that for this practice cash flow is not a problem and it would have no difficulty at all in raising the necessary funds to discharge its current liabilities. One could argue, however, that perhaps the practice is holding too much stock and that the cash in the bank would serve the practice better if it were invested.

If stock is taken out of the list of current assets, then the ratio of current assets minus stock to current liabilities for X and Y Veterinary Practice is around 5:1, which is still very good, but is a clearer indication that stock holdings are indeed too high. This ratio is called the *acid test ratio*, which it is argued is a better indicator of the liquidity of a business than the current ratio, because it may not be easy to convert stock into cash quickly. A veterinary practice needs its stock of drugs and medicines to function day to day and so cannot realistically dispose of all of it, but, conversely, too much stock means that cash which could be usefully utilized elsewhere by the practice or which could be earning interest is not available – admittedly, a debatable point given the current economic climate.

### Efficiency ratios

There are three key efficiency ratios which are used to measure how good the business is at managing stock, debtors and creditors. The *stock turn ratio* or *stock turnover ratio* calculates the number of times the entire asset of stock is sold during a financial year. To obtain this ratio, the opening and closing stock values are averaged:

(Opening stock + Closing stock) ÷ 2
    = Average stock

Then the cost of goods sold is divided by this average stock value to give the number of times per year that the entire stock holding is sold. Obviously, the higher the number, the better, because it shows that the business is not holding stock on its shelves too long and it is making more sales, which means that more income and more profit are being generated.

Cost of goods sold ÷ Average stock = X times

The '*debtor days*' ratio calculates the average number of days that the business takes to collect payment from its debtors. This is calculated using the following formula:

(Average debtors ÷ Total credit sales) × 365
= X days

The average trade debtors figure is calculated by taking the opening debtor figure (i.e. the balance of debtors at the start of a financial year), adding the closing debtor figure (i.e. the balance of debtors at the end of a financial year) and dividing the result by two:

(Opening debtors + Closing debtors) ÷ 2
= Average debtors

So, for example, if a practice's average debtor figure is £45,000 and the total credit sales for the period are £225,000, then this practice takes on average 73 days (approximately 2.5 months) to collect payment:

(£45,000 ÷ £225,000) × 365 = 73 days

Obviously, the quicker a practice can collect payment from debtors, the better, as a high debtor figure could negatively affect cash flow, so practices should work hard to keep debtors to a minimum.

'Creditor days' is calculated in a similar way, but using average creditor figures and total credit purchases. This ratio calculates the number of days the business takes to pay its creditors. Thus:

(Opening creditors + Closing creditors) ÷ 2
= Average creditors

(Average creditors ÷ Total credit purchases) × 365
= X days

So if a practice's average creditors figure is £65,000 and total credit purchases for the year are £565,000, then the practice takes on average 42 days to pay its suppliers:

(£65,000 ÷ £565,000) × 365 = 42 days

Generally, suppliers in the UK allow a maximum of 30 days' credit, so will not be very happy if a practice consistently pays after this time. There may be penalties for late payment and the practice could miss out on prompt payment discounts and other incentives. Relationships with suppliers also suffer if payment is not made in accordance with the terms agreed between the two parties, such that some suppliers may refuse to fulfil future orders.

These efficiency ratios are really more appropriate to businesses that engage solely in buying and selling stock (either bought in for resale or manufactured by them for sale to customers), and which generate significant numbers of debtors and creditors during

the normal course of their activities. Although veterinary practices also carry out these activities, they are not the primary activity of the practice, but rather are costs that arise from the provision of a service. Nevertheless, the principles represented by these ratios are relevant and it is still appropriate to calculate them.

### Investment ratios

Business owners invest their own money in the business and expect the business to provide a reasonable return on their investment. Most businesses are funded by a mix of money put into the business by the owners, a proportion of the profits earned and money that has been borrowed from the bank or other source. The Return on Capital Employed (ROCE) ratio expresses profit as a percentage of the total capital invested in the business. Total capital employed generally includes owner's capital, profits retained in the business (referred to as reserves) and long-term liabilities, such as loans. For X and Y Veterinary Practice (see Fig. 18.1), total capital employed includes the partners' capitals and capital account balances and totals £403,498. Profit before interest and tax amounts to £104,166. The ROCE is, therefore:

£104,166 ÷ £403,498 × 100 = 25.8%

which represents a good rate of return.

It is important that businesses do not rely too much on borrowed capital and long-term loans, but a certain amount of indebtedness is normal. 'Gearing' is a term in common use in accounting and refers to the level of borrowed capital that is being used to finance a business. There are several ways to calculate this ratio, but a simple method is to express the borrowings as a percentage of the total capital employed in the business. X and Y Veterinary Practice has a bank loan of £100,000. Total capital employed is £403,498, so the loan represents around 25% of all the capital utilized to run the business, which is a reasonable situation.

### Financial Performance Indicators (FPIs)

In addition to analysing financial data, practice owners need to regularly examine specific practice statistics obtained from activity and client data recorded using the practice management system. These statistics, also referred to as 'key performance indicators or KPIs', are an important performance monitoring and control tool, and often practice owners find them more meaningful and useful than accounting ratios.

A good practice management system should be able to output any type of raw financial data that a manager might want. The key, though, is to select the right data in order to generate a set of statistics that are useful, meaningful and helpful for decision making. Income data should be available directly from the system in ready usable form. Other statistics will need to be calculated, but spreadsheet software should help to automate this task once the raw data are transferred. Ideally, the computer system should produce reports either directly as Excel files or in a format that can easily be exported into a suitable software package of choice.

Table 19.1 lists a number of important statistics that practice managers will wish to monitor. The source of the data and the method of calculating these statistics are also given.

Monitoring practice income by income type enables managers to assess which activities generate the most income and which areas are the most profitable. Also, revenues generated from sales of drugs, medicines and pet products can be compared with revenues generated from the provision of services in order to ensure the optimal balance between the two. Ideally, a practice should be making most of its money from the provision of veterinary services in

which sales of drugs, medicines, food and pet products are generated by the service. The exact balance between the two types of revenue depends on the type of practice and the objectives of its owners.

Moreau and Nap (2010) emphasize the importance of closely following changes in client numbers. The numbers of active clients at the start and at the end of each financial year should be recorded, as well as the numbers of new clients registering during the year, numbers of clients who did not return and numbers whose pets have died. If these figures are monitored regularly, they allow the generation of some useful comparative statistics, which provide a strong indication of a practice's growth or decline. For example, a small animal veterinary practice started the year with 6500 active clients. During the year, 320 new clients registered, 250 clients did not return for reasons unknown and 150 clients' records were closed owing to pet deaths. Thus, at the end of the year, the number of active clients was 6420, representing an overall loss of 80 clients. This may only be a loss of around 1.23% of the practice's total client base, but if this downward trend continued in subsequent years, the loss would be cumulative. Of course, practice owners and managers will work hard to find out why clients leave so that they can prevent a decline in their client numbers. Interestingly, one could interpret the above statistic to mean that the practice has a client retention rate of 94% (client numbers at start of the year minus client losses during the year divided by initial client numbers), which might be viewed as an excellent retention rate but, in the longer term, if clients continue to be lost and are not replaced with new clients, this retention percentage will decrease.

The average transaction fee can be increased by either increasing prices or increasing the number of visits to the practice per client. Increasing client visits requires that the practice has something of value to offer in addition to what it is offering already, so it is important for practices to continue to look for new ways to satisfy client needs and to bring these to clients' attention. This will involve additional effort on the part of practice staff in terms of the development of new services and products and their promotion. If there is no slack in the system allowing time for this kind of activity, then it will be difficult to achieve. Increasing prices is obviously an easier alternative, but practices should beware of this course of action. Clients expect prices to go up each year but, as has already been

**Table 19.1.** Some important practice statistics.

| Statistic | Source/Calculation |
| --- | --- |
| Practice income, analysed month by month, into income types | Veterinary practice management system (VPMS) |
| Numbers of transactions, month by month | VPMS |
| Number of transactions per client | The total number of transactions divided by the total number of clients |
| Average spend per client | Total revenues divided by number of clients |
| Average transaction fee (ATF) | Total revenues divided by number of transactions |
| Average number of visits per client | Number of transactions divided by number of active clients |
| Net income per veterinarian | VPMS |
| New client numbers | VPMS |
| Active client numbers | VPMS |

argued, there is a limit to how much they are prepared to pay for services and products they consider to be optional or non-essential, or which they can get cheaper elsewhere. Then there is the competing practice down the road that always seems able to undercut. Price increases should ideally be accompanied by improvements in the standard of care and the tangibles that clients can see and experience – that way clients have clear evidence that their money is not simply disappearing into the owner's pocket, but that some of it, at least, is being returned to them through improved services.

## References

Dyson, J.R. (1994) *Accounting for Non-Accounting Students*, 3rd edn. Pitman, London.

Moreau, P. and Nap, R.C. (2010) *Essentials of Veterinary Practice: An Introduction to the Science of Practice Management.* Henston Veterinary Publications, Veterinary Business Development, Peterborough, UK.

Wood, F. and Sangster, A. (2002) *Frank Wood's Business Accounting 2*, 9th edn. Pearson Education, Harlow, UK.

## Revision Questions

**1.** Explain the difference between accounting ratios and KPIs.

**2.** A practice's debtors at the start and at the end of the financial year totalled £4500 and £6500, respectively. Credit sales for the year were £45,000. Calculate the debtor days ratio. What can you conclude about this practice's ability to collect payments from its debtors promptly? *(To check your calculations, refer to Appendix 3.)*

**3.** Why is it important to make comparisons with previous years as well as with industry norms for similar types of practice when assessing a practice's performance?

**4.** At the end of the financial year, a small animal practice had 6500 active clients on its books and the total number of transactions was 22,250. The practice decided that it would like to increase the overall number of transactions over the forthcoming year by 20%. Give two specific ways in which the practice might be able to achieve this.

# 20 Pricing Products and Services

Businesses that sell goods and/or services use a variety of methods in order to establish how much to charge their customers or clients. Veterinary practices are no different in this respect and there is no one correct method or formula that is used in the same way by all. The aim of this chapter is to explain the basic principles of pricing and to illustrate these by exploring the 'cost-based' and 'cost centre' methods of pricing products and services.

Veterinary practices engage in two types of business – the provision of services and the sale of products – two quite different offerings, but the basic principles of price setting can be applied to both in a broadly similar way. These principles are quite simple and can be summarized in the following way.

In order to ensure survival, the prices a practice charges for its work and for the products it sells must cover the costs of carrying out the work and for providing the products – it is as simple as that. Thus, in order to break even, income must equal costs. Survival may be a practice's primary aim, but in order to grow and develop it must make a profit. So the price to the client must also include a profit element.

## Costs

Before prices can be set, all the costs must be known. Parkinson (2007) defines 'cost' as a 'money-based measure of the resources used in order to generate outputs'. 'Resources' include things such as staff time, surgical materials, equipment, telephones, water, heating, lighting and so on. As has already been shown (Chapter 17), the 'Profit and Loss (P&L) Account' (also called the 'Trading and Profit and Loss Account') gives a summary of annual business costs. For pricing purposes, though, businesses need to enquire further about these costs – they need to know which costs can be directly attributed to a service or product being sold and which costs cannot. In order to make this important distinction, costs need to be grouped or 'sorted' into categories. The main method of sorting costs is to group them into *variable costs* and *fixed costs*. One can also group them into *direct* and *indirect costs*.

Variable costs are costs that vary as the volume of products sold or of services provided varies. So the more products that are sold or the more services that are provided, the more the variable costs will increase. For example, the number of bandages, disposable syringes or swabs used in surgery will increase the more operations are performed, and the overall cost of surgical consumables will increase accordingly. Fixed costs are costs that remain the same irrespective of the volume of sales or services provided. Examples of fixed costs are telephone rental, rent and insurances. The total cost of any product sold or any service provided will then include both variable and fixed costs, and before an accurate price can be set, it is necessary to identify and to assign a monetary value to these costs.

Direct costs are those that can easily and clearly be identified with a particular activity or product. Indirect costs cannot be identified with any activity or product and are often referred to as 'overheads' (Parkinson, 2007). So, when working out costs, overheads are either allocated to a particular activity or product or apportioned (shared) across a range of activities or products. From the foregoing, one might conclude that variable costs are the same as direct costs and that fixed costs are the same as overheads, and often that is indeed the case, but not always, depending on the activity. It is important to realize that these two methods of classifying costs are simply two different ways of looking at the same thing. In pricing veterinary products and services, the most common way of categorizing costs is into direct costs and overheads.

Direct or variable costs are relatively easy to identify as they are clearly associated with a

© C.R. Coates 2012. *Veterinary Practice Management* (C.R. Coates)

specific activity or product, but while we are able to name and list these costs, it is not always easy to assign a monetary value to them. Returning to the earlier example of the surgical removal of an intestinal foreign body from a 2-year-old Labrador bitch, we know that preoperative drugs are administered using a disposable syringe, that anaesthetic gases are administered throughout the operation, that disposable drapes, gowns and face masks are also used, as are cotton wool swabs, wipes and sutures, not to mention disinfectants, wound dressings and post-operative analgesics. The practice buys these consumables in and so will know their exact prices, but to price out every single consumable item used for every surgical procedure that the practice carries out would be a formidable task and one that is not usually undertaken as a routine. Because of the practical difficulties of establishing the exact costs involved in complex activities, managers responsible for setting prices will, of necessity, use methods which involve an element of estimation and guesswork. Thus, price setting is not an exact science. Nevertheless, it is essential that managers work to identify the costs as accurately as possible, as this will not only greatly assist in accurate pricing, but will also help to control costs by identifying those areas that are not as efficient as they should be.

## Pricing Products

The term 'products' refers to drugs, medicines, pet food, pet care products, baskets, beds, leads and toys – in other words, all items that the practice sells to clients in addition to the provision of a veterinary service. Practices generally buy in these items from drugs suppliers and wholesalers for resale to clients.

Over-the-counter pet care items are often supplied with a 'Recommended Retail Price' (RRP), at which the practice sells them. The RRP usually corresponds with the prices that can be charged for the same items by pet shops, supermarkets and other retail establishments. Because clients can easily obtain them cheaper elsewhere though, the profit that can be earned by a practice from their sale is minimal and practices have no choice but to apply a competitive sales price. Practices generally stock and sell these products mainly for the convenience of clients, and also because they often have the effect of encouraging clients to purchase other,

more profitable items. Ackerman (2003) argues that practices should not try to maximize profits on items to which no value is added – items that practices simply buy in and sell on without doing anything else with them. Nevertheless, it is important to ensure that all costs incurred in selecting, purchasing, storing and managing stocks of these items are recovered through appropriate pricing, otherwise they will be sold at a loss, which is unsustainable in the longer term.

Drugs and medicines for animal treatment are not usually supplied with an RRP. They are closely linked to the veterinary care provided and are prescribed by veterinarians who use their training and knowledge to select and recommend the appropriate medication for the pets under their care. Legislation governs the purchasing, storage, handling and supply of veterinary drugs and medicines. Therefore, the costs involved in providing them are greater and these must be recovered. However, even though the value-added component in the form of the veterinarian's expertise does justify price setting for profit, the profit element within the final price charged to the client must still be justifiable.

Even though clients are free to buy drugs and medicines from a range of alternative suppliers, as with other products, there are a number of excellent reasons why they should buy them from their veterinary practice and staff should be trained to explain these to clients whenever they raise a query about the price:

- The practice's drugs and medicines are always available in a form and at a dosage that is most appropriate for the patient.
- Veterinarians are familiar with the pet's history and are in the best position to answer questions about the administration, effects or side effects of the drugs or medicines they prescribe.
- Veterinary drugs and medicines are developed for specific species and specific medical conditions, so clients can be reassured that they are the most appropriate ones for their pets.
- There are strict controls on veterinary drug safety, drug quality and efficacy.
- Practices offer the convenience of a 'one-stop shop' to their clients so that they can obtain the necessary drug or medicine straight away rather than delaying treatment until they visit a pharmacy or until the drug arrives from an online store.

Ackerman (2002) suggests the following basic formula for working out the sales price of products:

Sales price = Fixed costs + Variable costs + Profit

Obviously, it would not be practical to try to work out the fixed and variable costs for every individual drug or medicine sold. A simpler method is to utilize the total annual expenses figures in order to work out the total annual cost. Some figures can be obtained directly from the P&L account, other costs will need to be worked out.

To illustrate, Fig. 20.1 shows a fictitious P&L account for a small animal veterinary practice.

In this practice, a veterinary nurse orders all the drugs and medicines and she spends 20 hours each week placing orders, resolving supplier queries, receiving deliveries, updating the practice stock database and restocking the shelves. An administrator checks the paperwork and processes supplier invoices. He has estimated that it takes him around 30 minutes each week to do this. Veterinarians also spend time reviewing current drugs stocks, researching new drugs and recommending new purchases and replacements. They estimate that this work takes around 1 hour of their time every week. They also spend time meeting with drugs company representatives and this takes up 2 hours of their time every 2 months.

Veterinarians also prescribe and dispense medications, but as this activity is dependent on the number of patients seen for whom medication is required, it is agreed that the cost in terms of veterinarian time involved will be recovered through a dispensing fee, to be added at the time the medicine is sold to the client.

The practice has a dedicated pharmacy, which occupies 1/30th of the practice space. The practice management system shows that £200 worth of stock was wasted, lost or damaged during the year. The pharmacy houses a large refrigerator, which cost £500 to buy 5 years ago and which will need replacing the following year. There is also a label printer in the pharmacy covered by a maintenance contract costing £25 p.a. The nurse cleans and tidies the pharmacy once a month and this takes around 2 hours each time. The nurse also carries out a full stock count once a year. This takes around 7 hours and is done during a weekend. The nurse receives 1.5 times her salary for this weekend work.

Taking into account the above information, and utilizing the figures in the P&L account given, pharmacy costs can be worked out as follows:

**Direct Variable Costs**

| | |
|---|---|
| Cost of drugs and medicines (opening stock + purchases – closing stock) | £223,960 |
| Losses/wastage | £200 |

*Staff Costs: Nurse*
Total nurse costs (salaries + pension + CPD) = £79,288 p.a.
Total hours worked p.a. = 4830
Cost per hour = £79,288 ÷ 4830 = £16.42
Cost of time spent on pharmacy = 126.5 h × £16.42 = £2,077

*Staff Costs: Veterinarian*
Total vet costs = £102,420 (Assistants × 2) + £49,500 (notional owner's salary) + £6,500 (pension costs) + £4,480 (locum fees) + £1,575 (travelling expenses) + £2,500 (CPD) = £166,975 p.a.
Total veterinarian hours worked p.a. = 4830
Cost per hour = £166,975 ÷ 4830 = £34.57
Cost of time spent on pharmacy = 58 h × £34.57 = £2,005

*Fixed Costs*

| | |
|---|---|
| Annual depreciation on refrigerator | £70 |
| Maintenance contract for label printer | £25 |
| Share of practice overheads: £305,297 ÷ 30 = | £10,177 |
| Total pharmacy costs for year: | £238,514 |

The practice's clients paid £358,000 for drugs and medicines, leading to a profit for the practice of £358,000 – £238,514 = £119,486, representing a markup on cost of approximately 50% and a profit margin of approximately 33.4%. Note that 'markup' is a percentage added to the cost price to give the sales price and 'margin' is profit expressed as a percentage of the sales price.

There are a number of issues that every practice owner and manager must consider when setting product prices and these are discussed in detail by Shilcock and Stutchfield (2008) and Ackerman (2002), but can be summarized as follows:

- A practice might expend considerable effort in trying to establish all the costs involved, but it is the market that ultimately determines the

## A Veterinary Practice
### Profit and Loss Account for the Year Ended 31st April 2012

| | £ | £ | £ |
|---|---:|---:|---:|
| Sales | | | 895,000 |
| *Less* Cost of sales: | | | |
| Opening stock | 40,000 | | |
| Purchases of drugs and medicines | 221,960 | | |
| Laboratory costs (internal) | 13,500 | | |
| Laboratory costs (external) | 22,100 | | |
| | 297,560 | | |
| Closing stock | (38,000) | | 259,560 |
| **Gross profit:** | | | **635,440** |
| | | | |
| *Less* Expenses: | | | |
| Surgical and anaesthetic consumables | | 26,230 | |
| Carcass disposal costs | | 9,950 | |
| Staff costs (Assistants × 2) | | 102,420 | |
| Staff costs (Nurses × 3) | | 75,108 | |
| Staff costs (P/T receptionists × 2) | | 25,036 | |
| Staff costs (Technician × 1) | | 17,070 | |
| Staff pension scheme | | 9,730 | |
| Locum fees | | 4,480 | |
| Travelling expenses | | 1,575 | |
| Vehicle costs (fuel, tax, MOT, repairs) | | 5,200 | |
| Rent | | 30,000 | |
| Council tax | | 9,500 | |
| Insurance | | 4,500 | |
| Heating and lighting | | 6,500 | |
| Repairs and renewals | | 16,250 | |
| Advertising | | 20,000 | |
| Stationery | | 12,500 | |
| Telephone and Internet | | 15,200 | |
| Mobile phones | | 1,080 | |
| Maintenance contract: computer system | | 5,650 | |
| Maintenance contracts: clinical equipment | | 6,500 | |
| Staff CPD (assistants) | | 2,500 | |
| Staff CPD (nurses) | | 950 | |
| Bank charges | | 10,200 | |
| Legal and professional fees | | 12,350 | |
| Bad debts | | 6,200 | |
| Depreciation | | 30,250 | |
| Interest on bank loan | | 15,825 | 482,754 |
| **Net profit** | | | **152,686** |

**Fig. 20.1.** A Profit and Loss (P&L) Account for a veterinary practice.

price, and practices often find it necessary to apply a range of different markups to match client expectations.

- Wholesalers and manufacturers often give discounts on the drugs and medicines that practices buy, which have the effect of lowering the cost to the practice. From an accounting point of view, supplier discounts are treated as income and the total of discounts received is added to gross profit in the trading and P&L account. It would only seem fair to pass on some of this benefit to clients in the form of discounts on relevant products. How much to discount, which products and for how long is up to the practice to decide.

- Drugs manufacturers and wholesalers increase their prices periodically and so it is necessary to regularly update the practice price list. Practice management systems are normally set up to automatically calculate the markup on cost price, but new prices have to be either manually entered on the system or uploaded from a supplier monthly price update disc.

- Where pharmacy cost calculations do not include the time spent by the veterinarian in selecting the appropriate medication, making decisions about dosages and amounts, dispensing, injecting or the costs of packaging and labelling drugs and medicines, it is reasonable to charge a small dispensing fee or injection fee in addition to the variable and fixed costs and profit.

## Constructing a Fee

The above method of working out pharmacy costs is referred to as 'cost-based pricing', which simply means identifying the costs involved in providing the products or services and then making an informed decision about how much to add for profit taking into account market pressures and competitor pricing.

Most practices base their fees loosely on cost. 'Cost centre analysis' is a cost-based method, which involves dividing the practice up into discrete areas in which similar types of activity take place and to which direct costs can clearly be allocated. Overheads costs are apportioned between these areas in various ways, either based on the floor area that they occupy or using other more appropriate methods, depending on what drives or causes a specific cost to arise. Thus a practice might be split into the following cost centres:

- Practice laboratory
- Radiology
- Anaesthesia
- Surgery
- Consulting (including health checks, vaccinations and outpatient procedures)

- Pharmacy
- Wards/hospitalization
- Office/administration.

A few direct allocations to cost centres can be made from the figures provided in the P&L account. For example:

| | |
|---|---|
| Internal laboratory expenses: | to Practice laboratory |
| Surgical consumables: | to Surgical suite |
| Maintenance contracts: clinical equipment: | to Surgical suite |
| Anaesthetic gases and consumables | to Anaesthesia |
| X-ray consumables: | to Radiology |

Staff costs include salaries, pension scheme, locum fees, travelling expenses for home visits and CPD costs. These costs are allocated to cost centres based on overall time spent within a cost centre or time spent completing a 'unit' of activity within a cost centre multiplied by the number of units completed during the relevant time period. Obviously, not all staff time will be spent on income-earning activity and this non-billable time will be included in the practice overheads.

The most accurate way to establish how much time is spent by staff on non-chargeable work is for staff to complete time sheets for a period of, say, 3 months, detailing all of their activities over that period. Unfortunately, for many practices this is simply not practical and so the time spent within the different areas of the practice and on specific activities will need to be estimated in the absence of such data. When allocating staff time to cost centres and to overheads, it is important to ensure that all staff costs are accounted for. In addition, if the practice owner is a veterinarian who works in the practice, but does not draw a salary, a 'notional' salary for them should be included in staff costs, based on what the practice would normally pay for this person if they were employed (see the total veterinarian costs calculated above). For the purposes of this example, it is estimated that veterinarians spend 68% of their time on fee earning activity and 32% on non-fee earning activity.

It should be possible to allocate carcass disposal costs to individual cases and thereby to pass these on directly to the client. A system should be put in place enabling the matching up of cremation costs with individual patients, but if this is not possible for some reason, these costs will need to be included in practice overheads.

The Office/Administration cost centre will be allocated stationery, computer maintenance contract costs and relevant staff costs. However, while it is important to know how much the administrative function costs the practice for cost-control purposes, the costs relating to this function will have to be apportioned across the cost centres that actually earn the practice money, otherwise this expense will not be covered by the fees charged.

The remaining costs, those that cannot be allocated to cost centres, are included in general overheads and will need to be apportioned across all the income-earning cost centres. General overheads will include the proportion of staff time that is spent on non-income earning activity.

Thus, taking the practice laboratory cost centre as an example, one might produce the following analysis:

**Variable Costs:**

| | |
|---|---|
| Reagent and materials costs: | £13,500 |
| Nurse's time: 84 h × £16.42 | £1,379 |

**Fixed Costs:**

| | |
|---|---|
| Depreciation of laboratory analyser: | £500 |
| Maintenance contract costs: | £217 |
| Proportion of practice overheads (£305,297 ÷ 60) | £5,088 |
| Total internal laboratory costs: | £20,684 |

If 600 laboratory tests are performed in a year, this would result in an average cost per test of £34.47. A suitable percentage for profit would be added to this to give the price to the client.

## Conclusions

Cost-based pricing and cost centre analysis are costing methods which enable a practice to identify and establish the costs associated with different activities. They provide managers with a range of different unit costs, which can be used to create the practice's price list. They also lead to a greater understanding of the costs of providing services and enable managers to review their fee structures from an informed position. Cost centre analysis, in particular, enables the identification of areas and activities that are not particularly efficient or profitable and allows managers to make changes to benefit the practice both in terms of efficiency and profitability. Clients also benefit, because prices are not set in an arbitrary fashion, but rather from a sound basis of real practice costs.

## References

Ackerman, L. (2002) *Business Basics for Veterinarians.* ASJA Press, Lincoln, Nebraska.

Ackerman, L. (2003) *Management Basics for Veterinarians.* ASJA Press, Lincoln, Nebraska.

Parkinson, A. (2007) Cost information. In: *B713 Fundamentals of Senior Management: Block 2 – Sessions 5–6.* The Open University, Milton Keynes, UK.

Shilcock, M and Stutchfield, G. (2008) *Veterinary Practice Management: A Practical Guide*, 2nd edn. Saunders Elsevier, Edinburgh, UK

## Revision Questions

1. Explain your understanding of the cost-based pricing method.
2. Using the figures given in the P&L account and your own estimates of direct costs and staff time required, calculate the annual cost of the Radiology profit centre. Assume that Radiology occupies 1/30th of the practice space.
3. The following costs are known:
    1 h veterinarian time = £35.65
    1 h nurse time = £15.00
    Surgical suite overhead portion = £25,650 p.a.
    Surgical and anaesthetic consumables costs = £26,230 p.a.
    Time spent in theatre by veterinarians in a year = 1360 h
    Equipment cost = £6,460 p.a.
Calculate the cost for an operation that lasts 1 hour and which requires one veterinarian and one nurse. (*To check your calculations, refer to Appendix 3.*)
4. How does cost-based pricing assist managers in making pricing decisions?

# SECTION 5
# Practice Growth and Development

**Section Objectives**

At the end of this section, you should be able to:

- Discuss the link between planning and business performance.
- Explain the process of strategic planning.
- Draft an outline business plan for your selected business.
- Explain payback, net present value (NPV) and internal rate of return (IRR) as methods of evaluating capital investments.
- Take an informed approach to managing projects.

# 21 Planning

Looking towards the future and setting goals is part and parcel of human existence. Similarly, in business, planning is a regular activity for business owners and managers. However, according to Orpin (2009), 'the conspicuous absence of a business plan is the norm for busy practices'. It is not that practice owners do not plan. On the contrary, they certainly have plans and generate ideas, but more often than not they fail to formalize them. In other words, plans are not documented or communicated to staff and there is no organized planning process in place. There are various reasons for this:

- Inertia – things appear to be functioning well without the need for planning.
- Perceived lack of time – owners and managers are often far too busy to spare the time.
- Perceived difficulty getting all the staff on board – it is often difficult to get all the staff together in the same place at the same time.
- Reluctance to put effort into preparing a written business plan, which may end up on a shelf gathering dust – owners and managers are well aware that planning is not a one-off activity.
- Lack of conviction of the benefits – there is little concrete evidence of the benefits of business planning.
- Fear of change – embarking on a planning process may well reveal that changes are needed.
- Lack of management training – owners and managers lack the knowledge and tools to enable them to plan effectively.

Around 81% of managers in large corporations routinely engage in business planning (Rigby, 2001, cited by Gibson and Cassar, 2005). These managers are obviously convinced of the benefits of planning for their own organizations. The link between performance and planning in SMEs, however, is less clear-cut. Schwenk and Shrader (1993) carried out a meta-analysis of 26 published studies examining the relationship between strategic planning and financial performance in small businesses and concluded that a positive relationship does exist between performance and planning, albeit a very subtle one.

Gibson and Cassar (2005) also examined previous studies and concluded that the causal relationship between planning and performance in small firms was at best inconclusive. They carried out their own longitudinal study over a period of 4 years in which data were collected from a large sample (2956) of Australian small firms (employing less than 200 staff). Their results did confirm a causal relationship between planning (in the form of documented business plans) and performance (as measured by sales and employment growth). The results also showed, however, that planning was more likely to be introduced into a business *after* a period of growth rather than before. Nevertheless, the authors observed that the more successful firms tended to be the ones that engaged in formal business planning. It appears, therefore, that formal planning is a routine management activity within the more successful SMEs, and certainly within these businesses it does appear to contribute towards sustaining business growth.

In order to establish the extent to which managers of SMEs think and act strategically, Stonehouse and Pemberton (2002) carried out research involving a sample of 150 manufacturing and service sector SMEs (mean number of employees 150) in the UK. Specifically, they wanted to find out the extent to which these businesses employed strategic planning tools and the degree of practical acceptance of the subject of strategic management. They found that the majority of the firms they studied recognized the importance of strategic planning and undertook formal planning, but kept their plans flexible, as circumstances dictated. Interestingly, their plans did not extend beyond 3 years, with one fifth of respondents operating a 1 year planning horizon, thus raising the question of whether such planning could actually be classed as strategic, because strategic planning is usually concerned with the longer term. The authors found that the majority of firms, particularly in the service sector, had clearly articulated mission statements and associated objectives, but when asked which specific planning tools they used, very few used typical strategic planning tools, such as STEP (also known as PEST – analysis of external sociological, technological, economic and political factors; or PESTLE – analysis of external political, economic, sociological, technological, legal and environmental factors) or Porter's Five Forces framework (Porter, 2008 and Chapter 16), preferring instead financial analysis, SWOT (strengths and weaknesses (internal), opportunities and threats (external)) analysis and benchmarking, which are more closely associated with operational planning. These findings are contradictory – on the one hand the firms surveyed appeared to appreciate that strategic planning was important, but when it came to the practicalities of implementing strategic planning, they retained a short-term focus and an operational planning approach; this suggested a fundamental lack of awareness of the need for longer term strategy and, possibly, a lack of knowledge or understanding of the strategic planning tools available. The authors point out that it is also possible, though, that the strategic planning tools may have been considered by the firms surveyed and subsequently rejected as not being relevant to them, although the research was unable to provide any evidence of this.

Although no research evidence is available about attitudes towards strategic planning in veterinary practices in the UK or the extent to which strategic planning tools are utilized by veterinary practice managers and owners, it is most likely that veterinary practice managers engage in similar forms of strategic planning to those outlined by Stonehouse and Pemberton (2002). There is also evidence of a growing interest in this area of management – and certainly no shortage of veterinary business advisors and specialists offering their services to practices who wish to undertake strategic planning for the first time.

## The Planning Process

Cole (2004) describes the planning process as managers defining 'ends' and identifying 'means' and 'conduct'. Thus, in order to plan, managers must have specific objectives in sight. The process begins, therefore, with defining aims and objectives (the 'ends'), then proceeds to identify the resources, both physical and human (the 'means') that are needed, and the processes, policies, actions and timescales (the 'conduct'), through which the objectives will be achieved. Cole (2004) points out the cyclical nature of planning – aims and objectives are continuously reviewed, and resources, processes and actions are changed or amended in light of the results achieved (Fig. 21.1). So planning is not something managers do once or twice a year and forget about in between, it is a continuous process of assessing outcomes and revising plans, while the overall business aims and objectives remain the same.

## Operational versus Strategic Planning

Most practice managers are involved with planning at an operational level, their main concern being the smooth functioning of the practice in terms of efficiency, deployment of human and physical resources, and ensuring quality of patient care and client service and the general day-to-day performance of the practice as a whole. Typical operational planning tasks are developing budgets, producing staff rotas, considering equipment needs, reviewing stocks or planning space utilization, among others. This type of planning tends to be limited to the short term, 1–2 years ahead at most.

Strategic planning determines the overall direction of a business and gives rise to operational planning. It concerns itself with the longer term, up to 5, perhaps even 10, years into the future, and seeks to place the business ahead of its competitors

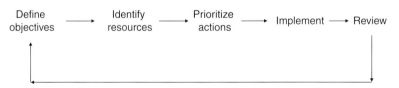

**Fig. 21.1.** The cyclical planning process.

Chapter 21

in order to establish a firm and lasting reputation with clients and other stakeholders. It is also about defining the business's mission, shaping its culture and ensuring continued growth and development. Vision and mission are translated into aims and objectives, which are, in turn, translated into specific goals and actions at the operational level. Strategic planning is normally the preserve of top management, and in veterinary practice one would expect the owners to take responsibility for this, but although they may be responsible for overall strategy, all staff will play their part in determining and, subsequently, achieving the aims and objectives that are set.

## The Strategic Planning Process

Strategic planning aims to address the following fundamental questions:

- Where do we want to be in 5–10 years' time?
- How do we get there?
- What are our prospects for growth and development?
- What resources will we need and how do we get them?
- What threats do we face now and in the future and what can we do about them?
- How is our operating environment likely to change and how should we respond?
- How can we gain an advantage over our competitors and maintain it?

In order to answer these questions, a three-stage process is undertaken:

**Stage 1.** Strategic data collection.
**Stage 2.** Strategic data analysis – building a picture of the practice to inform its future direction.
**Stage 3.** Strategic choice – defining vision and mission and overall strategy.

Once Stage 3 is completed, the overall strategy would then be translated into aims and objectives, actions and individual goals at the operational planning level.

### Stage 1. Collecting strategic data

The aim at this stage is to collect data in order to establish the practice's current position and circumstances and to identify future trends and changes that are likely to have an impact on the practice. Data are collected in four key areas:

1. *The external environment* – the influence of external environmental factors – a PESTLE analysis – data are obtained from the veterinary press, local and national news and media, government departments, such as Defra (the UK Department for Environment, Food and Rural Affairs), and other bodies to identify both current and future environmental influences and changes (see also the Introduction to this book).
2. *Clients* – their views of the service provided, their needs and interests both now and in the future – data are obtained from client surveys, a demographic analysis of the local population, local news, from talking to clients face to face and from practice–client focus groups.
3. *The practice's services and products* – obtained from an internal analysis of the practice's strengths and weaknesses, as part of a SWOT analysis. When assessing internal strengths and weaknesses, all areas of the practice should be reviewed – current financial position, the staff and their professional skills, premises and facilities, equipment and practice management system, current processes and procedures, and overall efficiency and effectiveness.
4. *Competitors* – the services they offer and their strengths and weaknesses – from their own brochures, web sites, advertisements and any promotional or PR activities they undertake.

The data collection process should be as objective and factual as possible, although a certain amount of 'crystal ball' gazing may be necessary when attempting to assess future trends and developments. If demographic or competitor data are difficult to obtain, it may be necessary to commission some market and competitor research, which will have to be paid for, but which is likely to be far more professional and thorough than the practice could achieve on its own.

### Stage 2. Strategic data analysis

The data obtained in Stage 1 are interpreted and organized in a way that will help to inform the future direction of the practice. The PESTLE analysis should reveal current and future developments taking place within the external environment, both near and far, that are likely to have an impact on the practice. Impending veterinary, employment or other legislation will be identified, requiring decisions about how to respond.

Client survey results should provide a clearer picture of client perceptions, future preferences and needs, and suggest ways in which the service could be improved or changed in order to meet these needs. Ideas for future services and facilities that could potentially be provided or different types of services and different approaches to service provision should also emerge.

SWOT analysis is a popular planning tool that is widely used by businesses and should give the practice a clearer idea of its internal strengths, which will support future plans, and its weaknesses, which are likely to prevent plans from being achieved unless something is done about them. The practice should also gain a clearer idea of external threats and any opportunities that it could potentially pursue.

A summary of findings for each area should be produced and written down, together with a list of actions emerging from the findings. No attempt at this stage is made to prioritize or organize the action list. These documents are then circulated to all staff and discussed widely. Staff could be asked to suggest priorities and put forward their own ideas of how the practice should proceed and how they see it developing over the next 5 to 10 years.

There are two specific tools that managers might find helpful at this stage – *critical success factor (CSF) analysis* and *scenario planning*. The first involves drawing on the data obtained to build a solid understanding of the environment, the industry and the practice itself, which then enables the identification of factors that are most *critical* to the success of the practice and ways in which these could be strengthened in order to ensure future success. Examples of CSFs might be:

- Clinical excellence
- High standard of patient care
- Client orientation
- Image and reputation
- Dedicated and motivated staff
- Flexibility and adaptability.

Having identified its CSFs, a practice would then consider strategies for their achievement or continued improvement.

Schoemaker (1995) describes 'scenario planning' as a 'disciplined method for imagining possible futures'. Utilizing the information obtained from the data collection process, managers build, say, a minimum of three alternative versions of the future in order to explore different strategic options that these would present. In doing so, they identify the ways in which the data interact (usually in a cause and effect relationship) and create stories around those interactions, which are then put together. Scenarios must be plausible, realistic and consistent. For example, a veterinary practice might come up with a scenario in which single-owner and partnership practices will no longer exist and where large groups and corporates will be the only veterinary business models in operation. In order to adapt to such a future, the choice might be either to join forces with two or more similar practices or to sell to a corporate within the next 5 years. In another scenario, the practice's immediate competitor might achieve veterinary hospital status and begin to offer a specialist internal medicine service in addition to first-opinion work. In order to compete, the practice might have to develop a similar capability, either in the same or in another discipline, or it might decide to excel at first-opinion work instead. Scenario planning is a useful tool for managers who are looking for new ideas, services or markets. If shared with staff and discussed widely, the scenario plans will draw on people's creativity and imagination and should generate further ideas. However, this tool is intended to be mainly informational and should not be used to dictate strategy.

### Stage 3. Strategic choice

Having collected the data and carried out their analysis, owners and managers should be ready to make a decision about the overall direction in which they want the practice to go. If the practice does not have a mission statement, they would formulate one with input from all staff. A mission statement is a succinct statement that expresses a business's core ideology and values and which provides a clear, focused direction. For example:

Our mission is to be the pet owner's first choice for veterinary services, delivering outstanding value through up-to-date skills and facilities and excellence in customer care.

Our mission is to continue to provide a first-class veterinary service to the pets in our care, to offer our clients modern, well-equipped premises staffed by committed, caring professionals.

A set of four or five broad strategic objectives are then set out, focusing on the specific areas which the practice wishes to develop. These objectives should be written in fairly general terms, but should be specific enough to allow an assessment of whether or not they are being achieved as time progresses. For example, if the practice decided to develop its exotics service as a referral service, a broad objective for this might be 'to grow a successful and profitable exotics referral service for veterinary practices in the South-West region', or if it decided to develop CPD courses for veterinary nurses, the broad objective for this might be 'to develop high-quality sought-after CPD courses for veterinary nurses'.

The broad objectives are then translated into specific, measurable objectives, which, in turn, are translated into goals for individuals and teams, who then formulate action plans and agree deadlines for the completion of the different stages and tasks involved. A detailed written business plan will specify the operational details for every aspect of the business covering the short term up to a period of 3 years. This plan should serve as a 'living document', which is revisited regularly and updated or amended, as necessary.

Regular progress reviews should be built into the plan, with the owners retaining overall responsibility for progress. The owners have a vital role to play in keeping the momentum going and ensuring that all staff remain motivated throughout the process. Once the work has started, the achievement of important milestones should be celebrated and successful individual contributions rewarded.

## Formalizing the Process

The process of strategic planning can be formalized by putting specific measures in place, such as:

- Creating a 'Practice Strategy' document containing the mission statement, the broad objectives, specific objectives and copies of plans with deadlines as developed by teams and individuals. This document should be disseminated to all staff, revisited regularly and kept up to date.
- Creating a business or operational plan covering the short term up to a period of 3 years, which is regularly reviewed and kept up to date.
- Holding regular progress review meetings, at least once every 3 months, in which everyone is required to report on progress to date, any difficulties encountered and, crucially, to

request assistance and/or resources needed to complete tasks.
- Including brief updates on the 'practice strategy' in general staff meetings.
- Holding 'celebration and reward' ceremonies when significant deadlines have been met and tasks completed.

## References

Cole, G.A. (2004) *Management Theory and Practice*, 6th edn. Thomson, London.

Gibson, B and Cassar, G. (2005) Longitudinal analysis of relationships between planning and performance in small firms. *Small Business Economics* 25, 207–222.

Orpin, P. (2009) Reaping the rewards of better management. *In Practice* 31, 84–87.

Porter, M.E. (2008) The five competitive forces that shape strategy. *Harvard Business Review* 86(1), January 2008, 78–93.

Rigby, D. (2001) Management tools and techniques: a survey. *California Management Review* 43, 139–160.

Schoemaker, P.J.H. (1995) Scenario planning: a tool for strategic thinking. *Sloan Management Review* 36(2), 25–40.

Schwenk, C.R. and Shrader, C.B. (1993) Effects of formal strategic planning on financial performance in small firms: a meta-analysis. *Entrepreneurship Theory and Practice*, Spring 1993, 53–64.

Stonehouse, G. and Pemberton, J. (2002) Strategic planning in SMEs – some empirical findings. *Management Decision* 40, 853–861.

## Revision Questions

**1.** Differentiate between 'operational' and 'strategic' planning and identify five specific management activities associated with each.

**2.** It is argued that strategic planning is of more use to businesses operating within a rapidly changing environment where there is a high level of uncertainty about the future. To what extent does your own experience lead you to agree with this argument?

**3.** Assess the types of planning that are undertaken in a practice with which you are familiar. How is this activity formalized?

**4.** Select one of the mission statements given in this chapter and write out four broad objectives that emerge from it.

# 22 Preparing a Business Plan

A business plan sets out a business's objectives and explains how and when these will be achieved (Barrow, 2001). It is an operational plan, which spells out the resources required and the operation of the business within each of the key areas of staffing, premises, physical resources, finance, marketing and organization. The business's marketing strategy is outlined, as well as how it intends to finance its plans. A well-written business plan will demonstrate that the managers' reasoning is sound and that all plans are backed up by financial evidence and plausible assumptions.

For an established business, a business plan forms part of its overall strategy for growth and development. For a new business, it serves as an important management tool for the owner as well as a means of persuading potential investors and lenders to invest in the business. Business plans map out a business in detail and, because of this, take a considerable amount of time and effort to prepare, but the processes involved, provided that they are undertaken thoroughly and with commitment, are of enormous benefit to owners and managers, because they teach them about their own business and help them to gain management knowledge and skills that they may not have had at the start. Lloyd (2007) argues that the primary aim of a business plan should not be to secure funding, but rather to develop a comprehensive picture of a business which is grounded in reality and based on disciplined decision making. Most experienced managers would agree that although a good business plan does not guarantee that a business will succeed in the longer term, it is an essential starting point for success.

There are numerous books available and plenty of information can be found on the Internet about how to write a business plan, together with details of what needs to be included in one. The aim of this chapter is to outline the main sections of a business plan and to discuss the contents of each. It is not the intention to provide specifics about how long the plan should be or how the document should be set out and presented, as this information is readily available elsewhere and depends completely on the type of business and the purpose for which the plan is being written.

## Components of a Business Plan

Most business plans will contain the following sections:

1. Executive Summary
2. Description of the Business and its Purpose
3. Management and Staffing
4. The Product(s) and/or Service(s) the Business Offers
5. Premises and Equipment (or Infrastructure)
6. Marketing Plan
7. Business Organization
8. Financial Projections
9. Appendices.

Logically, a manager will not begin writing before he/she has carried out the necessary research and obtained all the relevant information. Some of the research will mirror that which was outlined in the section on obtaining strategic data in Chapter 21.

## Executive Summary

The executive summary is a succinct summary of the business plan. Barrow (2005) refers to it as the 'essence' of the entire plan. Business advisors appear to agree that it should be written last, after the other sections of the plan have been completed. It is perfectly acceptable, however, to draft it out at the start and finalize it afterwards. Potential financiers will read this section of the plan first, and depending on whether it grabs their attention or not, will decide whether it is worth reading further.

Therefore, because it has such a decisive impact, the aim should be to make it as interesting and attention grabbing as possible, while taking care to avoid exaggeration. It goes without saying that it should put across a very positive picture of the business.

A good Executive Summary will be no more than two pages in length and will contain the following:

- A brief explanation of the reason for writing the plan – for example, if the purpose is to raise funds, state how much money is required, what this will be used for and what is offered to the investor in return. Or if the purpose of the plan is to map out the business's operational future as part of its longer term strategy, then state this and the period covered by the plan.
- Brief description of the management team and what makes them uniquely qualified to run this business – their skills, experience and knowledge that make them the ideal team to deliver what the plan promises.
- Description of the products and/or services being offered and why customers/clients will want them – how they differ from the competition and what makes them unique.
- The business objectives and the strategies for achieving them – a summary of the key objectives and how these will be achieved.
- Summary of the financial forecasts – brief summary of planned revenues and expenses and the level of profit the business intends to make.

## Description of the Business and its Purpose

For an existing business which is producing a business plan as part of a strategic planning exercise, this section describes the business's vision and mission and lists its key objectives. It is a good idea for managers to revisit these regularly. A business plan which is updated annually will help to ensure that they do this. Each key objective is broken down further into sets of goals and targets with timescales for the achievement of each one.

For a new business, this section describes the legal entity – whether a limited company, partnership, sole trader or other – the location of the business, head office address and web site domain name. The founder will also explain why this business is being formed. This is usually to fill a recognized

gap in the market, or to offer a new service for which there is a clear demand, or an existing product or service for which there is no supplier in the chosen area. Clearly, there must be a sound reason for setting up the business, resulting from thorough research and a knowledge of the market. The vision and mission are also outlined, together with the key objectives to be achieved over the next 3 years, thereby demonstrating that the founder knows exactly where the business is going. Key objectives will be translated into goals and targets and a realistic timescale for the achievement of these set out.

## Management and Staffing

This part of the business plan provides details of the individual(s) who will manage the business and the people who will be employed to work in it. Managers' unique experience and the skills and knowledge that make them ideally suited to run the business should be explained, with details of how these were acquired. The specific responsibilities to be undertaken by key staff and their roles within the business are discussed, specifically how each member will contribute to the business's success. Detailed CVs and job descriptions for key staff will be included in the appendices. Any plans for employing additional staff in the near future in order to fill skills gaps, or bring in additional labour as the workload increases, will be outlined, and the reasons given. If it is essential to a business's success that the staff should operate effectively as a team (and in which small business is this not essential?), then it is important to demonstrate that members bring complementary skills and are able to work effectively together and have done so successfully in the past. It is also important to demonstrate that an appropriate level of administrative support is available within the business, as well as professional and legal advice in the form of an accountant and a solicitor, and advisors to advise on HR and health and safety law (Stutely, 2007).

## Products and Services Offered

This section describes in detail the products and services being offered. If the intention is to offer a range of products and services, these should be listed and their importance to the business in terms of income share and contribution to profits should be explained.

An existing business may plan to offer one or two additional services or products and should explain these here, with the reasons why they are being offered. If existing services or products are being discontinued and replaced with new ones, then the reasons for this should also be explained.

A new business will not only describe the products and/or services being offered, but will also explain the way in which these differ from those of its direct competitors and why customers or clients would prefer them. If the product or service being offered is unique, then this should be pointed out and the nature of its uniqueness explained. It may be that the product or service is similar to that provided by other businesses, such as in veterinary medicine. If this is the case, there has to be something special about the service or product or the way in which it is delivered or in the additional benefits that the business brings to customers/clients that give it an advantage over its competitors and increase its chances of success. In veterinary practice, a unique location, few competitors in the area, a specialist service or extensive parking may provide the advantage required.

## Infrastructure

The infrastructure section concerns premises, equipment and other physical resources that the business will need to operate. Whether premises should be rented or bought outright depends on a variety of considerations – whether the founder has sufficient capital to buy, whether renting is the only option available or whether the option to purchase is available and realistic. Obviously, buying premises means that the business will own a considerable asset, despite the expense of having to pay a mortgage, but it may wish to sell at a later date and so the founder will need to choose carefully. Renting means that the business will be paying out money on a regular basis as an expense. There is no ready answer to this and the choice is up to the owner and will be dictated largely by circumstances. Once a decision is made, however, the choice of premises, the advantages of the location and reasons for the choice will be described here. It will be important to demonstrate that the chosen premises will accommodate all the activities of the business and allow for possible future expansion. If there is a lease, then the period of the contract will be given and any consequences of terminating the contract early outlined, should this be necessary at some stage.

This section will also contain a list of the major items of equipment that are already owned and of equipment that will need to be purchased, and how this will be used in order to generate revenues. Any items that confer a specific advantage, such as, for example, a standing MRI (magnetic resonance imaging) machine, which competitor veterinary practices do not own, should be described.

## Marketing Plan

Before this section can be written, some research needs to be carried out into competitors, customers and the environment within which the business intends to operate. Barrow (2005) insists that this is the most crucial part of the business plan as the marketing information obtained provides the foundation for financial projections, and these will not be convincing unless the marketing information is correct.

A start-up business will not have any customers or clients yet (or may have very few) and so will need to establish that there is a market for its products or services. The founders will either do the research themselves by devising and sending out their own questionnaire, for example, or, if there are funds, will commission it. The research should be targeted at the most likely customer segment and aim to establish whether there is a demand for the product or service being offered.

An established business will need to find out if its customers will still be there the next year and the next, as there are no guarantees, so it will be essential for the business to get to know its customers and correctly identify their needs so that the business can continue to ensure that these are met. Just how the business intends to do this in terms of promotional strategies employed will be outlined in this section of the plan.

For a start-up business, once potential customers have been identified, it is vital to ensure that the products or services offered match their needs as closely as possible, specifically that the benefits offered are what the customers want. Once this has been explained, the plan will then go on to describe the customer base and explain how the product being offered matches customer needs better than competitors' products. A plan for advertising and promoting the product or service will then be outlined, together with the associated costs.

Business owners should demonstrate a knowledge of their competitors and so some competitor research is essential. This is aimed at establishing who these competitors are, how many are there, how big they are and what their products are like. Information can be obtained from available databases, business directories or newspapers, or by drawing on the knowledge of friends and family. With veterinary practices, one way of finding out is to telephone a practice and ask for a brochure and price list. Inevitably, competitors will often be able to boast of greater strengths in some areas, but as long as a new business is able to demonstrate that it has effective ways in which it intends to compete, then it should be able to generate sales.

This section of the business plan will also contain an analysis of the external environment, of the impact of PEST (STEP) factors on the business and of how the business intends to meet the challenges and opportunities presented by these factors.

How much to charge for the product or service is both a marketing and a financial concern. On the one hand, any business must recover its costs and make a profit from the prices that it charges its customers. On the other hand, its prices cannot be so high that the customer will refuse to buy or so low that the customer will doubt the quality. Also, there are competitors' prices to consider. Most prices will be set based on a combination of cost and competitor pricing. Whichever pricing method is chosen should be explained and a rationale for the choice provided.

## Business Organization

This section concerns the supporting administrative systems that need to be in place to enable the primary function to operate. Thus, details of IT systems and of other record-keeping systems (e.g. client database, accounting), purchasing procedures, insurances required, and health and safety procedures will be outlined, with details of the ways in which these will support the primary function. The aim is to demonstrate that the underpinning systems are efficient, necessary and cost-effective, and that they fulfil all legal and legislative requirements. Any specific legislation that is relevant to the business and what it does will also be explained, together with the measures that have been put in place to enable the business to comply with this.

## Financial Projections

Forecast 'Profit and Loss (P&L) Accounts', 'Cash Flow Statements' and opening and closing

'Balance Sheets' should be provided for at least the first 2–3 years of trading. The P&L account and balance sheet have been explained elsewhere in this book. A cash flow statement is a summary of the movement of funds in and out of the business's bank account, showing literally the flows of cash into and out of the business. Cash is the life blood of any business, and so the business plan must show that there will be a healthy cash balance in the business's bank account at all times; in other words, that the owners know how to manage the business's cash so that it never runs out. In every business, there will be peaks when there is more money coming in than going out, and troughs, representing the opposite – with more money flowing out than in. The idea of good cash flow management is to anticipate and level off these peaks and troughs. A new business may well take some time before it starts to generate sufficient revenues to cover its costs and, therefore, it must ensure that it has a reserve of cash to cover this period.

The P&L accounts and cash flow statements are presented on a month-by-month basis rather than as summative, year-end accounts. Examples of these accounts for a fictitious single-owner veterinary practice are given in Tables 22.1 and 22.2.

It is customary to place these accounts in the appendix to the business plan and to simply detail the main points of the financial projections within the body of the plan. For both an existing business and a start-up business, the accounts represent a set of financial targets or budgets that they will work towards (Lloyd, 2007). However, while an existing business will have previous years' figures to compare with, it is extremely difficult for a start-up business to predict exactly how much income will be earned, as it really has limited information on how its customers will behave. Informed guesswork is often the only option, and projections will lie somewhere between the best and worst case scenarios. Arguably, costs are easier to predict. A business will list all of its anticipated costs and attempt a reasonable estimation. Overheads, such as rent, council tax, telephone line rental or insurances, can easily be estimated from figures supplied by the landlord and providers of these services. Direct costs of sales, or the variable costs that vary in line with the level of activity, may be more difficult to ascertain, but will be closely linked to the level of forecast sales.

**Table 22.1.** Example of a projected profit and loss (P&L) account for the first year of a fictitious start-up veterinary practice.

**A. Vet Limited**

Profit and Loss Projections for the Twelve Month Period Ending 31 March 2012

| | 2011 | | | | | | | | | 2012 | | | |
| | April | May | June | July | Aug | Sept | Oct | Nov | Dec | Jan | Feb | March | Totals F/Y |
|---|---|---|---|---|---|---|---|---|---|---|---|---|---|
| Sales | 6,500 | 6,260 | 5,845 | 4,320 | 4,100 | 6,500 | 10,250 | 13,888 | 14,660 | 15,450 | 16,100 | 16,720 | 120,593 |
| **Less Cost of Sales:** | | | | | | | | | | | | | |
| Opening Stock | 4,000 | 6,250 | 5,425 | 4,725 | 4,000 | 5,800 | 4,800 | 3,300 | 4,500 | 4,000 | 4,500 | 2,500 | 4,000 |
| Purchases (Drugs and Consumables) | 3,100 | 0 | 0 | 0 | 2,500 | 0 | 0 | 3,500 | 2,500 | 3,000 | 2,500 | 3,000 | 20,100 |
| Laboratory Fees | 450 | 420 | 400 | 400 | 395 | 460 | 650 | 675 | 695 | 695 | 700 | 720 | 6,660 |
| Clinical Waste Disposal | 350 | 330 | 310 | 310 | 300 | 320 | 556 | 650 | 675 | 675 | 712 | 750 | 5,938 |
| Casual workers/ Locums | 0 | 0 | 0 | 0 | 0 | 0 | 0 | 0 | 650 | 650 | 650 | 0 | 1,950 |
| *Less Closing Stock* | (6,250) (1,650) | (5,425) (1,575) | (4,725) (1,410) | (4,000) (1,435) | (5,800) (1,395) | (4,800) (1,780) | (3,300) (2,706) | (4,500) (3,625) | (4,000) (5,020) | (4,500) (4,520) | (2,500) (6,562) | (1,500) (5,470) | (1,500) (37,148) |
| **Gross Profit** | **4,850** | **4,685** | **4,435** | **2,885** | **2,705** | **4,720** | **7,544** | **10,263** | **9,640** | **10,930** | **9,538** | **11,250** | **83,445** |
| **Less Administrative Expenses:** | | | | | | | | | | | | | |
| Director's Remuneration | 462 | 462 | 462 | 462 | 462 | 462 | 462 | 462 | 462 | 462 | 462 | 462 | 5544 |
| Salaries and Wages | | 1,500 | 1,500 | 1,500 | 1,500 | 1,500 | 1,500 | 1,500 | 1,500 | 1,500 | 1,500 | 1,500 | 16,500 |
| Employer's National Insurance Contributions | 195 | 195 | 195 | 195 | 195 | 195 | 195 | 195 | 195 | 195 | 195 | 195 | 2,145 |
| Rent | 1,000 | 1,000 | 1,000 | 1,000 | 1,000 | 1,000 | 1,000 | 1,000 | 1,000 | 1,000 | 1,000 | 1,000 | 12,000 |
| Rates and Water | 108 | 108 | 108 | 108 | 108 | 108 | 108 | 108 | 108 | 108 | 108 | 108 | 1296 |
| Light and Heat | 250 | 250 | 250 | 250 | 250 | 250 | 250 | 250 | 250 | 250 | 250 | 250 | 3000 |
| Insurances | 208 | 208 | 208 | 208 | 208 | 208 | 208 | 208 | 208 | 208 | 208 | 208 | 2496 |

| | | | | | | | | | | | | | Total |
|---|---|---|---|---|---|---|---|---|---|---|---|---|---|
| Repairs and Maintenance | 2,250 | 3,000 | 2,000 | 450 | 200 | 200 | 200 | 200 | 200 | 200 | 200 | 200 | 9,300 |
| Telephone Costs | 100 | 100 | 100 | 100 | 100 | 100 | 100 | 100 | 100 | 100 | 100 | 100 | 1200 |
| Postage and Stationery | 400 | 550 | 234 | 234 | 234 | 234 | 234 | 234 | 234 | 234 | 234 | 234 | 3290 |
| Equipment Hire | 0 | 0 | 0 | 0 | 0 | 0 | 0 | 320 | 320 | 320 | 320 | 320 | 1600 |
| Subscriptions | 61 | 61 | 61 | 61 | 61 | 61 | 61 | 61 | 61 | 61 | 61 | 61 | 732 |
| Advertising | 2,800 | 250 | 250 | 250 | 250 | 250 | 250 | 250 | 250 | 250 | 250 | 250 | 5,550 |
| Motor and Travel Costs | 307 | 307 | 307 | 307 | 307 | 307 | 307 | 307 | 307 | 307 | 307 | 307 | 3684 |
| Sundry | 300 | 300 | 300 | 300 | 300 | 300 | 300 | 300 | 300 | 300 | 300 | 300 | 3600 |
| Consumables | | | | | | | | | | | | | |
| Accountancy Fees | 200 | 200 | 200 | 200 | 200 | 200 | 200 | 200 | 200 | 200 | 200 | 200 | 2400 |
| Bank and Card Charges | 188 | 188 | 188 | 188 | 188 | 188 | 188 | 188 | 188 | 188 | 188 | 188 | 2256 |
| Depreciation | 450 | 450 | 450 | 450 | 450 | 450 | 450 | 450 | 450 | 450 | 450 | 450 | 5400 |
| **Total Expenses** | **9,084** | **9,129** | **7,813** | **6,263** | **6,013** | **6,013** | **6,013** | **6,333** | **6,333** | **6,333** | **6,333** | **6,333** | **81,993** |
| **Net Profit/Loss** | **-4,234** | **-4,444** | **-3,378** | **-3,378** | **-3,308** | **-1,293** | **1,531** | **3,930** | **3,307** | **4,597** | **3,205** | **4,917** | **1,452** |

Table 22.2. Example of a cash flow projection for the first year of a fictitious start-up veterinary practice.

**A. Vet Limited**

**Cash Flow Projections for the Twelve Month Period Ending 31 March 2012**

| | | 2011 | | | | | | | | | 2012 | | | |
|---|---|---|---|---|---|---|---|---|---|---|---|---|---|---|
| | | April | May | June | July | Aug | Sept | Oct | Nov | Dec | Jan | Feb | March | Totals F/Y |
| **Cash Inflow:** | | | | | | | | | | | | | | |
| Receipts from Clients | inc. VAT | 7,800 | 7,512 | 7,014 | 5,184 | 4,920 | 7,800 | 12,300 | 16,665 | 17,552 | 18,540 | 19,320 | 20,064 | 144,671 |
| Shareholders' Investment | | 0 | 50,000 | 0 | 0 | 0 | 0 | 0 | 0 | 0 | 0 | 0 | 0 | 50,000 |
| **TOTAL RECEIPTS** | | 7,800 | 57,512 | 7,014 | 5,184 | 4,920 | 7,800 | 12,300 | 16,665 | 17,552 | 18,540 | 19,320 | 20,064 | 194,671 |
| **Cash Outflow:** | | | | | | | | | | | | | | |
| Drugs and Consumables | inc. VAT | 3,720 | 0 | 0 | 0 | 0 | 3,000 | 0 | 0 | 4,200 | 3,000 | 3,600 | 3,000 | 20,520 |
| Laboratory Fees | inc. VAT | 0 | 540 | 540 | 480 | 480 | 474 | 552 | 780 | 810 | 834 | 834 | 840 | 7,164 |
| Clinical Waste Disposal | inc. VAT | 0 | 420 | 396 | 372 | 372 | 360 | 384 | 667 | 780 | 810 | 810 | 854 | 6,225 |
| Casual Workers/Locums | | 0 | 0 | 0 | 0 | 0 | 0 | 0 | 0 | 650 | 650 | 650 | 0 | 1,950 |
| Director's Remuneration | | 462 | 462 | 462 | 462 | 462 | 462 | 462 | 462 | 462 | 462 | 462 | 462 | 5544 |
| Salaries and Wages | | | 1,500 | 1,500 | 1,500 | 1,500 | 1,500 | 1,500 | 1,500 | 1,500 | 1,500 | 1,500 | 1,500 | 16,500 |
| Employer's National Insurance Contributions | | | 195 | 195 | 195 | 195 | 195 | 195 | 195 | 195 | 195 | 195 | 195 | 2,145 |
| Rent | | 3,000 | 0 | 0 | 3,000 | 0 | 0 | 3,000 | 0 | 0 | 3,000 | 0 | 0 | 12,000 |
| Rates and Water | inc. VAT | 648 | 0 | 0 | 0 | 0 | 0 | 648 | 0 | 0 | 0 | 0 | 0 | 1296 |
| Light and Heat | inc. VAT | 0 | 0 | 0 | 804 | 0 | 0 | 804 | 0 | 0 | 804 | 0 | 0 | 2412 |
| Insurances | | 2621 | 0 | 0 | 0 | 0 | 0 | 0 | 0 | 0 | 0 | 0 | 0 | 2621 |
| Repairs and Maintenance | inc. VAT | 0 | 2,700 | 3,600 | 2,400 | 540 | 240 | 240 | 240 | 240 | 240 | 240 | 240 | 10,920 |

| | | | | | | | | | | | | | | Total |
|---|---|---|---|---|---|---|---|---|---|---|---|---|---|---|
| Telephone Costs | inc. VAT | 0 | 0 | 0 | 360 | 0 | 0 | 360 | 0 | 0 | 360 | 0 | 0 | **1080** |
| Postage and Stationery | inc. VAT | 0 | 440 | 605 | 281 | 281 | 281 | 281 | 281 | 281 | 281 | 281 | 281 | **3574** |
| Hire Purchase Payments | inc. VAT | 0 | 0 | 0 | 0 | 0 | 0 | 0 | 0 | 384 | 384 | 384 | 384 | **1536** |
| Subscriptions | | 732 | 0 | 0 | 0 | 0 | 0 | 0 | 0 | 0 | 0 | 0 | 0 | **732** |
| Advertising | inc. VAT | 3,360 | 0 | 300 | 300 | 300 | 300 | 300 | 300 | 300 | 300 | 300 | 300 | **6,360** |
| Motor and Travel Costs | | 0 | 307 | 307 | 307 | 307 | 307 | 307 | 307 | 307 | 307 | 307 | 307 | **3377** |
| Sundry | inc. VAT | 0 | 360 | 360 | 360 | 360 | 360 | 360 | 360 | 360 | 360 | 360 | 360 | **3960** |
| Accountancy Fees | inc. VAT | 0 | 0 | 0 | 0 | 0 | 1440 | 0 | 0 | 0 | 0 | 0 | 0 | **1440** |
| Bank and Card Charges | | 0 | 188 | 188 | 188 | 188 | 188 | 188 | 188 | 188 | 188 | 188 | 188 | **2068** |
| VAT | | 0 | 0 | 0 | 0 | 0 | 0 | 800 | 0 | 0 | 2840 | 0 | 0 | **3640** |
| **TOTAL PAYMENTS** | | **14,543** | **7,112** | **8,453** | **11,009** | **4,985** | **9,107** | **10,381** | **5,280** | **10,657** | **16,515** | **10,111** | **8,911** | **117,064** |
| **NET INFLOW/ OUTFLOW** | | **−6,743** | **50,400** | **−1,439** | **−5,825** | **−65** | **−1,307** | **1,919** | **11,385** | **6,895** | **2,025** | **9,209** | **11,153** | **77,607** |
| Opening Bank Balance | | 0 | −6,743 | 43,657 | 42,218 | 36,393 | 36,328 | 35,021 | 36,940 | 48,325 | 55,220 | 57,245 | 66,454 | |
| Closing Bank Balance | | −6,743 | 43,657 | 42,218 | 36,393 | 36,328 | 35,021 | 36,940 | 48,325 | 55,220 | 57,245 | 66,454 | 77,607 | **77,607** |

For a start-up business, the figures should show a reasonable increase in revenues over the period covered and should demonstrate that the business will reach a position of profit within the stipulated time frame. All assumptions that were made when preparing the figures should be clearly explained, as they will not be self-evident to the reader.

## Conclusions

A business plan describes a business in detail and outlines its objectives for growth and development. The process of developing a business plan teaches managers about their business and about the challenges they face in terms of gaining clients, competitor advantage, external environmental threats and opportunities, and the practicalities of day-to-day operations. In identifying and analysing these, managers are able to define business direction and develop strategies that will enable their businesses to survive and prosper.

It is the nature of business plans that they have a limited 'shelf life'. What was valid and reasonable at the time the plan was prepared may no longer be the case a year on. Thus, it is essential that business plans are revisited regularly and kept up to date if they are to serve the purpose for which they are intended – as a road map for a future that is constantly changing.

## References

Barrow, P. (2005) *The Best-Laid Business Plans, How to Write Them, How to Pitch Them*. Virgin Books, London.

Lloyd, D. (2007) *Business Plans*. Hodder Education in Association with the Chartered Management Institute, London.

Stutely, R. (2007) *The Definitive Business Plan – the Fast-Track to Intelligent Business Planning for Executives and Entrepreneurs*, 2nd edn (revised). Pearson Education, London.

## Revision Questions

1. Explain where the business plan fits into an existing business's strategic plan.
2. Why is a written business plan essential for a start-up business?
3. Describe the business planning process in terms of the business knowledge required to run a business.
4. Examine the P&L and cash flow forecasts and explain the key differences between them.

# 23 Evaluating Capital Investments

From time to time it will be necessary for a practice to make capital investments – to fund a new enterprise, or a business expansion, or buy expensive items of equipment, either to replace existing equipment that has become obsolete or because of a perceived urgent need. Sound management principles require practice owners and managers to evaluate (or appraise) such investments in terms of their associated risks and potential financial return. Most businesses do not have the luxury of being able to spend large sums of money on a whim, even though this may occasionally happen if a salesperson is very convincing about the benefits of a particular item and the temptation is too great!

Whenever an investment of any magnitude is made, a business must assess the risk of doing so. Other factors also come into play in determining whether to make the investment or not. For most businesses, there are two key factors (Girotti, 2008):

- The effect on cash flow – is there enough cash available to fund this, should it be an outright purchase or would a lease arrangement be preferable?
- The rate of return – can the business make an adequate return on this investment and, if so, when will the benefits become available?

In the case of large items of equipment, these do not need to be purchased outright if cash flow is critical. There are various lease and hire purchase options available, which may be more expensive in terms of total overall outlay, but which can be beneficial, because:

- Any negative effects on cash flow are minimized.
- They can bring tax advantages.
- Risk is reduced or retained by the leasing company.
- Warranties and servicing are built in.

Some lease arrangements will allow the business to purchase the equipment at the end of the term of the lease; others may provide replacement equipment after a certain period of use. Leasing means that the equipment is never owned by the business, but is merely 'hired', so the leasing company carries the entire risk if the equipment malfunctions. This is a sensible option if the equipment has high maintenance costs, will be used only occasionally, or has a short useful life. With a hire purchase agreement, the business makes regular payments and once all the payments have been made, it will eventually own the asset (Business Link, 2012), so this method of financing is a means of spreading the cost of purchase.

## Risk and Uncertainty

From a business point of view, investing in new equipment or in a new project is only really worthwhile if the owner can be certain that the benefits will outweigh the costs. The benefits do not necessarily have to be financial as long as the owner is satisfied that they are sufficiently worthwhile. The difficulty lies in accurately ascertaining both benefits and costs. Some costs and benefits will be known and others will have to be estimated, and it is not always possible to do so with an acceptable degree of accuracy.

If the intention is to earn extra revenues from the investment, then predictions about future returns will have to be made, even though there can be no certainty that these will actually be earned. If the only option is to fund the investment or project with borrowings, the cost of the repayments may increase unexpectedly if interest rates rise at a later date.

In making the decision whether to go ahead with an investment or project, managers will undertake a 'risk analysis' and attempt to assess the impact of different levels and types of risk on the viability of the project. For example, things could go wrong with the business's internal processes, which may have a negative impact on the revenues it was hoping to generate from the new item of equipment or project. A significant change in any one of the external PESTLE factors could affect the level of demand, the price that can be charged or the availability of clients wanting the new product or service. Obviously, managers will not attempt to assess all of the conceivable risks, but only those that are relevant to the specific investment being proposed.

Of course, there is always going to be uncertainty and risk in any new investment or undertaking. The question is whether managers are prepared to go ahead knowing the level of risk and whether they consider this level of risk to be acceptable.

Another important point that must be borne in mind is the fact that the value of money changes over time, so £10,000 today will have a much lower value in the future. Consequently, any future returns will need to be discounted by applying an appropriate discount rate, which, once again, is an estimate based on the cost of capital and the perceived level of risk. The cost of capital relates to the interest rate payable on loan capital or the level of return an investor would require if they invested in the project.

## Methods of Evaluating Capital Investments

There are a number of different methods of evaluating capital investments, some more useful than others. The appraisal of any investment should be undertaken using several different methods of analysis rather than just relying on one. Different methods have their advantages and disadvantages, but when used together should result in useful information that enables managers to make a more informed decision.

As a starting point, two basic analyses could be undertaken: those for the accounting rate of return (ARR) and payback. Neither of these takes account of the time value of money or of risk, and so they are rather simplistic methods of limited usefulness, but they are often used, because they are easy to understand.

To illustrate, let us assume that an equine veterinary practice wishes to purchase a portable, battery-powered digital X-ray machine costing £15,000. This would be a new addition to the practice and the practice manager has calculated that it will

generate around £9500 extra income, because more X-rays will be performed. It is estimated that the machine will have a useful life of around 6 years, after which time it will have a residual value of £3000. The annual depreciation is £2000. The service contract on the machine costs £500 per year.

### Accounting rate of return (ARR)

The ARR simply compares the average annual revenue generated with the amount of the investment and expresses the revenue (minus depreciation) as a percentage of the amount invested:

$$ARR = \frac{Revenue - Depreciation}{Captial\ invested} \times 100$$

Thus, the investment in the portable X-ray machine gives an ARR of:

$$ARR = \frac{£9500 - £2000}{£15,000} \times 100 = 50\%$$

A value of 50% is good for an ARR. The higher the ARR, the more attractive the investment.

### Payback

Payback simply divides the amount invested by the anticipated annual revenues, and gives the period of time it will take for the investment to be recovered.

Thus, the payback period on the X-ray machine is:

$$Payback\ period = \frac{£15,000}{£9500} = 1.58\ years$$

### Net present value (NPV)

Two methods of appraisal that take into account the time value of money and the level of risk involved in an investment or a project are the net present value (NPV), discussed here, and internal rate of return (IRR), discussed in the next section. In order to appraise an investment using these methods, estimates need to be made of all the *cash* inflows and outflows of the investment over its entire lifetime. Because these estimates are made using the present value of money, the net inflow/outflow for each year of the investment is calculated and then discounted using a discount rate, which is selected to reflect the cost of capital and the level of risk. Discounting, then, reduces the net future values for each year to their present-day equivalent values. Deciding on what discount rate to apply is problematic, however, and there are no rules for this. It is advisable, therefore, to assess the investment using two or three different discount rates – a low rate reflecting low risk, and a higher rate reflecting higher risk. Tables showing the value of £1 discounted over varying numbers of years using different discount rates are available to download from the Internet.

Thus, assuming the practice buys the machine outright, the NPV calculation for the X-ray machine using a discount rate of 10% is as follows:

| Year | 0 | 1 | 2 | 3 | 4 | 5 | 6 |
|---|---|---|---|---|---|---|---|
| Capital cost | (15,000) | | | | | | |
| Revenues | | 9,500 | 9,500 | 9,500 | 9,500 | 9,500 | 9,500 |
| Service contract | | (500) | (500) | (500) | (500) | (500) | (500) |
| **Net cash flow** | (15,000) | 9,000 | 9,000 | 9,000 | 9,000 | 9,000 | 9,000 |
| Discount factor | 1 | 0.91 | 0.83 | 0.75 | 0.68 | 0.62 | 0.56 |
| **Present value** | (15,000) | 8,190 | 7,470 | 6,750 | 6,120 | 5,580 | 5,040 |

giving

NPV = –£15,000 + £8190 + £7470 + £6750 + £6120 + £5580 + £5050 = £24,150

This is a positive result, suggesting that the X-ray machine will be a sound investment. The actual amount arrived at is not as relevant as the fact that the NPV is positive. The calculation is based on some erroneous assumptions – that the revenues will remain the same year on year and that there will be no additional costs other than the service contract, which, again, is assumed to remain the same. Clearly, this will not be the case in reality. The general rule with the NPV is, therefore, to make the investment if the NPV is greater than zero and not to make it if the NPV is less than zero. A positive NPV suggests that the investment or project will earn at least the cost of capital used to pay for the investment.

A discount rate of 20% would result in the following NPV calculations:

| Year | 0 | 1 | 2 | 3 | 4 | 5 | 6 |
|---|---|---|---|---|---|---|---|
| Net cash flow | (15,000) | 9,000 | 9,000 | 9,000 | 9,000 | 9,000 | 9,000 |
| Discount factor | 1 | 0.83 | 0.69 | 0.58 | 0.48 | 0.40 | 0.34 |
| Present value | (15,000) | 7,470 | 6,210 | 5,220 | 4,320 | 3,600 | 3,060 |

giving

NPV = –£15,000 + £7470 + £6210 + £5220 + £4320 + £3600 + £3060 = £14,880

This is still a positive result.

### Internal rate of return (IRR)

The rate of return that is expected to be earned on the capital invested in a project is called the internal rate of return. The IRR is equivalent to the discount rate that would result in an NPV of zero. If the IRR percentage is greater than the cost of capital, then it is worth making the investment. Working out the IRR involves a ridiculously complex formula, which will not be explained here. As an alternative method, it is possible to search the present value tables for a discount rate that would give the desired result, but this could take some time. The simplest method is to use the IRR facility in Excel, in which the Excel IRR formula is applied to the present value figures for each year that have been input (in the present example those for years 0 to 6). In this example, the IRR is 42% for a discount rate of 10% and 30% for a discount rate of 20%.

### Payback using discounted cash flows

It is argued that payback calculations provide a more accurate estimate of the time that it would take for the initial investment to be recovered if discounted cash flows are used, so using the discounted cash flow figures instead, the payback period is as follows:

| Year | Cumulative cash inflows | Investment minus inflow |
|------|------------------------|-------------------------|
| 0    |                        | (15,000)                |
| 1    | 8,190                  | (6,810)                 |
| 2    | 15,660                 | 660                     |
| 3    | 22,410                 | 7,410                   |
| 4    | 28,530                 | 13,530                  |
| 5    | 34,110                 | 19,110                  |
| 6    | 39,150                 | 24,150                  |

At the end of Year 1 there was still £6810 outstanding on the investment. If annual revenues are £9000, then the amount outstanding will take (£6810 × 365) ÷ £9000 = 276.18 days to pay back. Therefore, the total payback period is 1 year and 276.18 days or 1 year and 9.08 months, which is longer than the initial payback calculation of 1.58 years made earlier.

## Conclusions

Payback and ARR are simple methods of capital investment appraisal, which are useful for gaining a general idea of whether an investment or project is worth undertaking or not. These methods should be supplemented by more sophisticated and reliable methods, such as NPV and the IRR, which are perhaps somewhat over the top for a relatively small investment such as the X-ray machine purchase used as an example in this chapter, but for larger investments, they are suitable methods for ascertaining whether it is worth going ahead or not. However, all of these methods have shortcomings, based as they are on estimates of future revenues, profits and cash flows, the reliability of which can be questioned. NPV and IRR assume, for the sake of simplicity, that all cash flows occur at the end of a period, which is not the case. None of the methods takes into account taxation or inflation, which are important external factors that can have a significant impact on business cash flow.

## References

Business Link (2012) Decide whether to buy or lease assets. Available at: http://www.businesslink.gov.uk/bdotg/action/layer?topicId=1073959001 (accessed 7 June 2012).

Girotti, R. (2008) Avoiding white elephants in capital expenditure. *In Practice* 30, 344–347.

## Revision Questions

1. When considering investing in a new piece of equipment, why should a manager use investment appraisal techniques instead of simply relying on their experience and 'gut feeling', which have worked well for them in the past?

2. Explain the concept of 'risk' and speculate about the potential risk factors in the external environment that could have a significant impact on the success of a new small animal orthopaedic referral service which a practice wishes to launch.

3. A practice is considering purchasing a new laser surgery unit at a cost of £25,000. It has estimated that the unit will bring in £5500 in extra revenues in year 1, increasing by 20% annually for the next 5 years. The service contract on the unit will cost £650 a year. The practice will take out a loan to buy this unit at an annual cost of 10%. Calculate the net present value (NPV) and advise the practice manager whether the practice should go ahead with this investment or not. Note that the discount factors for each of year 1 to 6 for a discount rate of 10% are given in the chapter. *(To check your answer, refer to Appendix 3.)*

4. Explain your understanding of internal rate of return (IRR) as an investment appraisal technique.

# 24 Managing Projects

A 'project' can be defined as a one-off substantial task or set of tasks which must be completed in order to achieve a specified objective within a defined timescale. From time to time practice managers may be called upon to manage projects. Whether it is a move to new premises, setting up a new service or facility, or carrying out a practice reorganization, they may find themselves responsible for organizing and overseeing the entire process and all the staff involved in it. Projects might be short or long term; they may take several months or several years to complete and are usually undertaken in addition to a manager's normal duties. Project management demands a combination of organizational, communication, leadership and administrative skills to ensure that the project is completed on time, to budget and to the standards required by the sponsors – whether that is the boss or another business or organization that has commissioned the project and is putting up the funds.

For some time now, the skill of project management has been recognized as a discipline in its own right and there are a number of courses and course providers in the UK that deliver the necessary training. A well-known project management standard is PRINCE 2 (PRojects IN Controlled Environments), a de facto standard which is used extensively by government departments and within the private sector. Irrespective of the PRINCE 2 standard, however, there is no one single correct way to manage a project. In the absence of specific training, individual managers will establish their own methods based on what works best for them within their own context. Larger organizations often devise their own protocols and procedures and train their managers to follow these.

The aim of this chapter is to examine the key stages of a project and to provide guidance on the management of each stage. Before proceeding, however, it is useful to explore what is already known about the factors that contribute to or that hinder a project's success.

A successful project can be defined as a project that has achieved its objective(s) within the budget and timescale specified and to the required standard. Elbeik and Thomas (1998) reviewed a number of large-scale projects and discovered that those which had failed shared the same shortcomings:

- The project objectives were unclear.
- Objectives were only partially achieved.
- The stipulated timescale was not adhered to.
- The stipulated budget was exceeded.

White and Fortune (2002) surveyed project managers who collectively identified three criteria, which they used to judge project success: successful projects are completed on time, to budget and to specification. The managers also judged project success against their perceptions of the degree of fit between the project and the organization, and the impact of the project on the business's overall performance. Following on from these key criteria, the managers identified four top-ranking factors as being critical to project success:

- Clear objectives
- Realistic timescale
- Sufficient resources (both human and physical)
- Support from senior management.

Thus, in the experience of project managers, if these four key things are properly attended to, then the chances of success are considerably enhanced.

Munns and Bjeirmi (1996) make a clear distinction between the project itself and project management as a tool for handling 'novel or complex activities'. Their definition of a project accords with the definition already given, but also mentions that projects consume resources and have definite start and end dates. Project management, in contrast, is defined by Munns and Bjeirmi as a process of controlling the achievement of project objectives, which utilizes a range of tools and techniques and which defines the work that needs to be done, allocates resources, plans, monitors progress and makes adjustments to deviations from the plan. The authors cite current literature which suggests that project success is dependent on a list of factors, but that only two of these – definite and realistic goals and the implementation process – lie within the scope of project management. For Munns and Bjeirmi, project management definitely plays an important role in project success, but is itself affected by other factors, which are not under the direct control of the project manager and which can cause a project to fail. The authors suggest that successful project management is characterized by:

- A commitment to complete the project
- A skilled project manager
- Time taken to define the project objectives adequately
- Effective planning
- Effective communication.

To increase the chances of success, therefore, project managers need to possess a degree of skill but, more importantly, should be aware of the factors that are known to contribute to project success and should ensure that these are properly attended to within the projects that they are responsible for.

## The Project 'Life Cycle'

Projects proceed through a series of identifiable stages from conception through to implementation, completion and, finally, closure or handover. Once a project is completed, it is useful to evaluate the process in order to learn from it and take forward important lessons for any future projects.

The key stages of a project can be listed as follows:

- Pre-planning
- Planning
- Implementation
- Monitoring and Control
- Completion and Evaluation.

Most projects will not progress through these stages sequentially, but will do so iteratively – in other words, planning will continue throughout the life cycle of the project, as will monitoring and control. Project objectives may be amended and timescales changed as a result of control decisions.

Thus, a certain amount of backtracking will inevitably occur, but as long as the work proceeds in the right direction, this is acceptable.

## Pre-planning

Most projects are preceded by a feasibility study, the aim of which is to establish whether the project is worth undertaking or not. The feasibility study will include a preliminary assessment of the resources required – those that are already available and those which will need to be brought in – timescales, stakeholders and their interests, and a financial appraisal of costs and returns using the methods described in Chapter 23 and others. The feasibility study is often written down as a formal document for presentation to the board or management team and is instrumental in the decision whether to proceed with the project or not. Because of its importance, every feasibility study should be carried out as thoroughly as possible and be based on objective data that are as accurate as possible. As part of the feasibility study, managers will also assess the consequences of not going ahead with the project.

If the decision is made to proceed, a project team is appointed. In a veterinary practice, the project 'team' generally consists of the practice manager, co-opted members of staff and, if used, outside contractors who may be carrying out the majority of the work. It is essential that all the stakeholders in the project are involved from the start and that effective communication channels are set up to ensure that everyone is kept appropriately informed of developments throughout the duration of the project.

At this stage, the budget is agreed and personnel who will be authorized to spend against it are identified. Risk assessments are carried out in order to identify any risks associated with completing the project, particularly those involving external contributors, such as contractors, suppliers or movers. An assessment is made of what is likely to go wrong and the impact of these eventualities, and contingency plans devised in order to minimize delays and unforeseen occurrences, which can have expensive consequences. A number of measures can be taken at the outset to protect against the consequences of things going wrong, such as setting up written agreements with contractors and suppliers, taking out special insurance policies or obtaining professional advice on legal issues or health and safety before proceeding.

Once the preparatory work has been completed, it is advisable to write down the key details of the project in the form of a 'project brief', which represents the 'terms of reference' to be referred to throughout the implementation stage. The project brief will contain the following information:

- Start and end dates
- Key objectives
- Key targets and deadlines
- Names and roles of the project team
- The budget
- Resources, both human and physical, that are to be utilized
- Reporting lines and decision-making protocols
- Communication arrangements.

Detailed timescales will be decided upon at the planning stage and can be inserted into the project brief once known (Martin, 2007).

## Planning

The project plan is a detailed breakdown of the work that needs to be done. It should show all the tasks and activities, their sequence and timing, the individuals responsible for completing them and the resources needed. Some of the tasks and activities can be carried out concurrently and others may only be completed sequentially – in other words, the first task must be completed before the next one can begin. A tool that is particularly useful for planning is a logic diagram. A simple logic diagram can be easily created using Post-it notes and a whiteboard. The Post-its are labelled with the key work stages and then placed in sequence on the whiteboard between the 'start' and 'finish' labels. Arrows are drawn to link the Post-its and to show the dependencies between the tasks. When drawing logic diagrams, the following conventions should be adhered to:

- The diagram flows from left to right.
- Timescales are not decided yet.
- The duration of each task is not relevant at this point.
- Different coloured Post-its should be used for different activity groups.
- The position of each note in the diagram should be debated until everyone agrees.
- Tasks should not be assigned to people yet.
- The diagram should be transcribed on to paper and a record of decisions made should be kept.

To illustrate the principle, let us assume that a practice manager and his team are given the task of producing a publicity brochure promoting the practice's new state-of-the-art kennelling facility. The intention is to distribute the brochure to pet stores, shops and local businesses in the area. Figure 24.1 shows a logic diagram that the project team came up with following discussion.

The logic diagram represents the skeleton of the plan, which now needs fleshing out. Each key stage identified should be broken down into tasks and lists of tasks should be drawn up. At this point, task duration, start and finish dates, and who will carry out each one can be decided and agreed upon. It is essential to secure the agreement and commitment of everyone involved when deciding on tasks, because task ownership will increase staff motivation to complete the project.

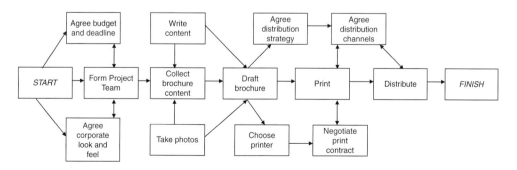

**Fig. 24.1.** A simple logic diagram for the production of a publicity brochure.

Once all the tasks have been identified, a task schedule is produced. A popular tool for this purpose is a Gantt chart which, in its simplest form, is a grid that plots the tasks, listed in sequence, down the left-hand side of the grid, against days and weeks that progress across the grid. Symbols can be inserted at specific points in the grid to show key events, such as team meetings, or key deadlines. Such charts can be created using project software such as Microsoft® Project or Primavera Project Planner®, but Excel can serve just as well. An extract from the Gantt chart produced for the brochure project is given in Fig. 24.2.

The 'critical path' is the sequence of tasks that would enable the project to be completed in the shortest possible time taking into account key dependencies: places where some tasks cannot commence until others are completed first. It is important to mark the critical path in the project schedule, either using arrows or a different colour font for relevant tasks, so that they stand out.

There are several different software packages that are specifically designed for project management and these can be useful, especially for complex, multistage and multitask projects. However, managers must beware of overcomplicating the task schedule, which is easy to do using sophisticated software, because they then run the risk of creating a schedule that others may not be able to understand or follow.

## Implementation

Implementing the plan means carrying out the agreed tasks in accordance with the task schedule. The project manager will be responsible for keeping the momentum going and the staff motivated. The manager must also ensure that everyone knows what is expected of them, that they have the necessary resources and that they know who to approach in the event of difficulty, especially if they are unable to meet the deadlines set for whatever reason. Progress meetings must take place regularly and staff should expect to attend and report on the progress they have made to date.

If individual progress is dependent on others, delays may occur while individuals wait for others to complete their parts of the project. This can cause resentments, and relationships to deteriorate, if not properly handled. Expectations should be made clear at the outset, and the consequences of delays and disruptions caused for reasons that could easily be avoided must be spelt out, so that everyone is clear about the impact of their actions or inaction on others. If it is possible to build in some form of reward system or a promise of a big celebration at the end, if the project is completed successfully, on time and to budget, then this can act as a motivator and keep everyone on track.

The project manager must also bear in mind that project work is often additional to staff's usual duties and will inevitably put additional pressure on them. Depending on how critical the project timescales are, it may be necessary to release individuals from their usual duties to enable them to complete their part of the project on time. Thus, the project manager needs to be aware of workloads and have a backup plan in place to provide the necessary flexibility at critical stages.

| Task Number/ Code | Description | Duration in weeks | Wk 1 6 Feb | Wk 2 13 Feb | Wk 3 20 Feb | Wk 4 27 Feb | Wk 5 5 Mar | Wk 6 12 Mar | Wk 7 19 Mar | Wk 8 26 Mar | Wk 9 2 Apr |
|---|---|---|---|---|---|---|---|---|---|---|---|
| A1 | Form Project Team | 2 | | | | | | | | | |
| A2 | Agree tasks | 1 | | | | | | | | | |
| A3 | Agree responsibilities | 1 | | | | | | | | | |
| A4 | Agree meeting frequency | 1 | | | ♦ | | | | | | |
| B2 | Research printers | 2 | | | | | | | | | |
| B3 | Research distribution | 2 | | | | | | | | | |
| B4 | Agree printer contract | 2 | | | | | | | | | |
| C1 | Write content – JD, AB, CC | 3 | | | | | | | | | |
| C4 | Photographs – CC, ST | 2 | | | | | | | | | |
| D1 | Collate content – JD, AB | 3 | | | | | | ♦ | | | |
| etc | | | | | | | | | | | |
| ♦ Team meeting | | | | | | | | | | | |

**Fig. 24.2.** Example of a simple Gantt chart created using Microsoft® Excel.

From time to time, it may be necessary to alter the plan for reasons outside a manager's control. Provided that appropriate contingency plans are in place and some degree of flexibility is built in, this should not cause the project to fail, even though it may delay its completion. Whenever this occurs, it is important to keep a written record detailing the causes of the delays and what was done about them. This record will be useful later on at the evaluation stage.

## Monitoring and Control

Throughout the implementation stage, the project manager will be continuously monitoring progress, making decisions and taking appropriate action. He/she will be comparing progress with the plan and identifying any actions that need to be taken in order to ensure that the project continues to progress as it should. Inevitably, not everything will go according to plan and adjustments will need to be made. One thing that a manager can do to keep everyone on track is to keep in touch informally with those involved in the work by visiting them and having brief 'catch-up' talks to check that everything is progressing smoothly. Informal contact, provided that it is not too frequent or too controlling, will enable the manager to resolve any day-to-day issues that might arise straight away rather than waiting for a progress meeting to take place. It is important for those carrying out the work to know that the manager is interested in them, is supportive and values their contribution. This will help to maintain staff motivation.

## Completion and Evaluation

Large-scale projects will have a handover schedule and there will be set criteria for the management of the handover process. But even with smaller projects, it is a good idea to have some kind of formal handover and acknowledgement of completion. This could be just a final report by the project team made at a staff meeting, followed by thanks expressed by the boss; or a formal opening of a new building with an invited celebrity and special guests; or a final meeting of the project team followed by a party. The format will very much depend on the type of project and the circumstances, but what is important is that the successful completion of a project is celebrated and that staff contributions are properly acknowledged, as this will greatly enhance morale.

After the celebrations have taken place, it is a good idea to carry out a post-mortem on the project outcomes, along with a final check that all the tasks have been completed and that there is no further work to be done. The project evaluation should include an assessment of the following:

- All paperwork associated with the project – this should be fully accounted for, labelled and filed safely for later retrieval, if required.
- The project timescales – whether these had been adhered to and, if not, the reasons for the delays and how they could have been avoided.
- The project budget – was the project completed to budget? If not, what was the extent of the overspend and how will this be recovered?
- What went well and not so well and what lessons have been learnt for the future?
- The key stages of the project – were they completed as planned?
- The contribution of the project to the success of the business as a whole.
- The contribution of the project to staff development.

It is advisable to produce a final written report detailing the findings of the evaluation. This should be as factual as possible and should avoid placing blame on anyone. It is important to ensure that it is read and agreed by everyone involved in the work so that the lessons for any future projects are learnt by all.

## Conclusions

Project management is a management discipline in its own right and the necessary skills can be learnt. The planning principles outlined in this chapter are relevant not only to project management, but also to anyone who has a substantial task to complete and needs to plan this out before proceeding – whether it is a research-based dissertation, a career plan or a work project. The approach described can help to clarify objectives at the start, will aid effective time management and will maximize the chances of success.

## References

Elbeik, S. and Thomas, M. (1998) *Project Skills*. Butterworth-Heinemann, Oxford, UK.

Martin, V. (2007) Preparing a project. In: *B713 Fundamentals of Senior Management, Block 4, Session 1*. The Open University, Milton Keynes, UK, pp. 7–52.

Munns, A.K. and Bjeirmi, B.F. (1996) The role of project management in achieving project success. *International Journal of Project Management* 14, 81–87.

White, D. and Fortune, J. (2002) Current practice in project management – an empirical study. *International Journal of Project Management* 20, 1–11.

## Revision Questions

1. Describe the key stages of the project 'life cycle' and give three rules for the management of each stage.

2. During the implementation stage, what is the project manager's primary concern and why?

3. List five ways in which the project manager can monitor the progress of a project.

4. Explain why it is important to carry out an evaluation of a completed project.

# SECTION 6
# Forms, Templates and Checklists

These documents can be adapted for use in practice, as required. Students are advised to study them and become familiar with their contents, layout and purpose.

- Appraisal Meeting Checklist
- Appraisal Process Checklist
- Job Description Template
- Job Vacancy Shortlisting Record and Guidance Notes
- Person Specification Template
- Staff Induction Timetable
- Template for Developing New Protocols and Procedures.

# Appraisal Meeting Checklist

1. **Review of performance over the review period**
   - (a) Job description ❑
   - (b) Review last year's targets ❑
   - (c) Training and development undertaken ❑
   - (d) Specific achievements ❑
   - (e) Issues and/or problems ❑
   - (f) Facilitators and barriers ❑
   - (g) Agenda discussion ❑

2. **Plan future performance**
   - (a) Discuss appraisee potential and future plans ❑
   - (b) Agree targets ❑
   - (c) Identify training and development needs ❑
   - (d) Identify resources, equipment, other needs ❑
   - (e) Agree plan of action ❑
   - (f) Write down action plan ❑

3. **Summarize discussion** ❑

# Appraisal Process Checklist

1. Start of process        Date: ...............
   (a) Notify all staff    ❏
   (b) Distribute forms    ❏
   (2 weeks)       Date: ...............

2. Appraisee and appraiser exchange forms, comment, agree agenda    ❏
   (2 weeks)       Date: ...............

3. Set date and time for appraisal meetings    ❏
   Organize location    ❏

4. Appraisal meetings take place    ❏
   (*timing dependent on number of staff to be appraised – aim to complete all meetings within 1 month of exchange of forms*)

5. Appraisers write reports and send to appraisees    ❏

6. Appraisees receive reports and amend/comment    ❏

7. All reports completed and signed off    ❏

8. Paperwork collated, checked and filed    ❏

9. Collect staff feedback on process    ❏

10. Carry out process review    ❏

11. Analyse results and identify actions    ❏

12. Report on process review to principal and staff    ❏

13. Actions resulting from review completed    ❏

Forms, Templates and Checklists

# Job Description Template

<Practice Logo>

<Practice name>
<Practice address>
<Contact tel. number(s)>
<Web site URL>
<E-mail address>

**Job Title**
**JOB DESCRIPTION**

| | |
|---|---|
| **Background Information** | About the practice – its aims, vision and mission, staffing, facilities and equipment and general ethos and culture |
| **Overall Purpose of the Job** | Succinct paragraph about the importance of the job and how it contributes to the goals of the practice |
| **Location** | Where is the postholder going to be working? |
| **Working Hours and Any Out of Hours (OOH) Requirement** | Specific details about working hours, working times, rotas and the OOH requirements |
| **Salary Range** | Specify not only the range, but also if salary is negotiable or not and, if so, what this depends on |
| **Reporting Lines** | Who does the postholder report directly to? Does anyone report to the postholder? |
| **Duties and Responsibilities** | A list of the main duties and responsibilities |
| **Scope** | Details of how 'big' the job is in terms of budgets managed, numbers of orders processed in a week, numbers of clients seen in a day, average numbers of hospital inpatients responsible for, etc. |
| **Additional Duties** | List any duties that should be completed, but which are outside the main purpose of the job, e.g. accompanying practice manager to the bank once a week, or delivering food and drugs orders to disabled clients, etc. |
| **Development and Promotion Opportunities** | If available, detail what promotion and development opportunities the practice offers |
| **Training Provided** | Detail any CPD (continuing professional development) allowance that is available and any training that is specifically provided, i.e. health and safety (including fire safety) training, induction training, training to use the practice management system, etc. |

# Job Vacancy Shortlisting Record

**CONFIDENTIAL**

<Practice Logo>

<Practice name>
<Practice address>

**Job Vacancy Shortlisting Record**

| Job Title | |
|---|---|
| Ref. Number | |
| Date Advertised | |

| No. | Applicant Name | Online application? Y/N | Reject – Give Reason (see guidance notes) | Interview (please tick) |
|---|---|---|---|---|
| | | | | |
| | | | | |
| | | | | |
| | | | | |
| | | | | |
| | | | | |
| | | | | |
| | | | | |
| | | | | |
| | | | | |
| | | | | |
| | | | | |
| | | | | |
| | | | | |
| | | | | |
| | | | | |

Signed: ...............          Date: ...............

See Guidance Notes on p. 2.

page 1

## Job Vacancy Shortlisting Record: Guidance Notes

This is a formal record of your decisions regarding which applicants to invite for interview and which to reject. All the paperwork relating to the post will be kept on file for a minimum of 6 months from the date of completion of the selection process.

Please ensure that you carefully consider each application and assess it against the job description and person specification documents you have been given. Any decision to reject an application should be explained by using one (or more) of the codes given below. At this stage you should not confer with other staff involved in the selection process, as short-listing decisions should be taken independently.

Please return your completed form to the Practice Manager/Principal. The deadline for completion of this process is ................

The results from the short-listing process will be notified to you and a list of applicants to be invited for interview will be provided no later than one week after the short-listing process together with interview information.

**Codes:**

II = Insufficient information provided in the application to enable suitability for the post to be determined

QI = Qualifications inadequate or unsuitable for the position

EI = Insufficient experience

SI = Skills inadequate for the post

KI = Insufficient knowledge

O = other reasons – *please specify*

page 2

# Person Specification Template

*<Practice Logo>*

<Practice name>
<Practice address>
<Contact tel. number(s)>
<Web-site URL>
<E-mail address>

Job Title
PERSON SPECIFICATION (or CANDIDATE PROFILE)

|  | Essential | Desirable |
|---|---|---|
| 1. Academic Qualifications | List all the essential educational qualifications that the ideal candidate should possess, e.g. GCSEs, A levels, degree, etc. | List any additional educational qualifications that would be useful. |
| 2. Professional Qualifications | List the essential professional qualifications required for the post. | List any additional professional qualifications that would be useful. |
| 2. Knowledge | What do you expect the candidate to know for the job? | What else might be useful for the candidate to know? |
| 3. Skills | Skills sought which are not specifically covered by the professional qualification, but which are essential. | Detail any additional skills that would be useful for the post. |
| 4. Experience | List the relevant experience that the ideal candidate would possess. Specify the type of other, additional experience required. | Detail any other type of experience that would be useful for the post, but is not essential. |
| 5. Supervisory Experience | If relevant, detail the supervisory experience the ideal candidate would possess – either in terms of numbers and types of staff supervised or in terms of types of supervisory experience possessed. | |
| 6. Personal Qualities | Detail personal qualities sought, such as communication skills, team working, flexibility, etc. | Detail any additional qualities that might be useful. |
| 7. Other Skills Required | Detail any additional skills that are being sought which are not covered elsewhere in the person specification, e.g. holder of clean driving licence. | Detail any additional extra skills that would be useful. |

# Staff Induction Timetable

<Practice logo>
<Practice name>

Staff Induction Timetable

| Information/Training | Date Completed | Signature of Line Manager/ Supervisor |
|---|---|---|
| **Week 1, Day 1 – Welcome to the Practice by Practice Principal/Practice Manager** | | |
| Practice Manager – complete paperwork, i.e. P45/P46, NI number, bank details for salary payments, Receive ID/security card and Staff Handbook and sign receipt | | |
| Introduction to 'buddy'/'mentor' | | |
| Tour of practice with 'buddy', including location of own office, equipment, toilet facilities, meal and refreshment arrangements and rules for clinical areas, staffroom, staff notice board | | |
| Introduction to Line Manager and key members of practice staff | | |
| **Week 1, Day 1 – Security: Line Manager** | | |
| Security alert status levels | | |
| Telephone system and bleep system | | |
| Security and safety protocols | | |
| Emergency procedures | | |
| Door keypad entry numbers, as applicable | | |
| Staff responsibilities – reporting lines | | |
| **Week 1, Day 1 – p.m.** | | |
| Reading/private study | | |
| **Week 1, Day 2 – Health and Safety Briefing: Practice Safety Advisor** | | |
| Practice health and safety policy | | |
| Codes of practice | | |
| Local rules and fire drills | | |
| COSHH (control of substances hazardous to health) assessments | | |
| Accident reporting procedure and location of first aid kits | | |
| First aiders | | |
| Risk assessments specific to the job | | |
| Protective clothing | | |
| Medicines and controlled drug (CD) cupboard protocols | | |
| Out-of-hours (OOH) safety procedures | | |
| VDU operating guidelines/workstation assessment | | |
| Disposal of sharps and clinical waste procedures | | |

| | | |
|---|---|---|
| **Week 1, Day 2 – Introduction to Radiologist** | | |
| Briefing on radiation hazards/X-ray no-go areas | | |
| Complete form for X-ray badge | | |
| Tutorial on the use of X-ray equipment – as applicable | | |
| **Week 1, Days 3–5** | | |
| Familiarization with requirements of the job with 'buddy' | | |
| **Week 1, Day 5 – p.m.** | | |
| Review of first week's induction with Line Manager | | |
| **End of Week 1 Induction Training** | | |
| **Week 2, Day 1 – Review of Job Description – Duties and Responsibilities: Line Manager** | | |
| Written terms and conditions issued | | |
| Contract of employment issued | | |
| Clarification of specific duties and responsibilities as outlined in job description and any questions arising from Week 1 | | |
| Arrangements for continuing on-the-job support and training | | |
| Line management and reporting structures operational in the practice | | |
| Policies on flexible working, time off in lieu, overtime payments | | |
| Probationary period | | |
| Performance appraisals – frequency and procedure | | |
| Private use of e-mail, the Internet and telephone policy | | |
| Holiday arrangements | | |
| Sickness reporting procedure and record keeping | | |
| Discipline, grievance and appeals procedures | | |
| OOH work | | |
| Clarification of work systems and procedures – *finish reading Handbook* | | |
| Ordering stationery and general office consumables | | |
| Office equipment requirements | | |
| Claiming expenses and fees | | |
| Training allowances | | |
| System for ordering consumables, drugs, medicines – procedures and responsibilities | | |
| IT facilities – e-mail, intranet, practice web site | | |
| **Week 2, Days 3–5 – Job Familiarization** | | |
| 'Buddy' assistance, as required | | |
| **Week 2, Day 5 – p.m. Review of Induction Process: Line Manager** | | |
| Review topics covered – identify any gaps and make arrangements to fill these | | |
| Review the process and identify any improvements that could be made | | |
| Review checklist completion and sign off | | |

**To be completed by new member of staff:**

Except for the subjects crossed out as not being applicable to me, I have received information and guidance as outlined in this timetable.

Signed: ...............             Date: ...............

**To be completed by Line Manager:**

The above member of staff has received induction training and guidance as indicated on this timetable.

Signed: ...............             Date: ...............

*THIS TIMETABLE SHOULD BE RETURNED TO THE PRACTICE MANAGER WHEN COMPLETED AND WILL BE KEPT IN THE EMPLOYEE'S PERSONNEL FILE*

# Template for Developing New Protocols and Procedures

TEMPLATE FOR DEVELOPING PROTOCOLS AND PROCEDURES

1. Define the protocol/procedure, why is it needed? Why is it important?

.................................................................................................................................

.................................................................................................................................

.................................................................................................................................

.................................................................................................................................

.................................................................................................................................

.................................................................................................................................

.................................................................................................................................

.................................................................................................................

2. List the actions that should be included in the protocol/procedure (i.e. what needs to be done)

.................................................................................................................................

.................................................................................................................................

.................................................................................................................................

.................................................................................................................................

.................................................................................................................................

.................................................................................................................................

.................................................................................................................................

.................................................................................................................

3. Who should be involved and in what way? (Must all staff comply? Are there specific roles and responsibilities that should be allocated?)

.................................................................................................................................

.................................................................................................................

..........................................................................................................
..........................................................................................................
..........................................................................................................
..........................................................................................................
..........................................................................................................
.................................................................................................

**4. How will the protocol/procedure be recorded? Does it need to be written down?**

..........................................................................................................
..........................................................................................................
..........................................................................................................
..........................................................................................................
..........................................................................................................
..........................................................................................................
..........................................................................................................
.................................................................................................

**5. Who will write it?**

..........................................................................................................
..........................................................................................................
..........................................................................................................
..........................................................................................................
..........................................................................................................
..........................................................................................................
..........................................................................................................
.................................................................................................

**6. Where will this document be kept and how will staff access it?**

..........................................................................................................
..........................................................................................................
..........................................................................................................
..........................................................................................................
..........................................................................................................

......................................................................................................

......................................................................................................

.............................................................................................

7. Who is going to keep the protocol up to date and keep staff informed of any changes?

......................................................................................................

......................................................................................................

......................................................................................................

......................................................................................................

......................................................................................................

......................................................................................................

......................................................................................................

.............................................................................................

8. What will be the consequences of non-compliance?

......................................................................................................

......................................................................................................

......................................................................................................

......................................................................................................

......................................................................................................

......................................................................................................

......................................................................................................

.............................................................................................

9. How often should this be reviewed and updated?

......................................................................................................

......................................................................................................

......................................................................................................

......................................................................................................

......................................................................................................

......................................................................................................

......................................................................................................

.............................................................................................

# Appendix 1
# Computer Terminology Explained

MICHAEL W. COATES

## Hardware and Software

The PC itself, as well as cabling, monitors, keyboards, mice and any other peripherals, are examples of hardware. Hardware alone however, is not particularly useful. To make use of the computer and other physical devices, software is necessary. Software contains the instructions required to control the hardware in order to accomplish the tasks required by the user. Software takes the form of programs, which are lines of code written by developers in a programming language, such as C or C++. Programs are written on to a CD or DVD disk or can be downloaded from the Internet.

Normally, a piece of software is designed to operate on a particular type of computer. In the early days of business computing, there were many different platforms, which were incompatible with each other, so that software written for one type of computer 'platform' would not work with any other and, frequently, data stored on one type of computer could not easily be read by another. Since the early 1980s, however, the IBM Personal Computer (hence PC) spawned several 'compatibles' – computers made by brands other than IBM that could use the software written for the PC. Mainly because of this, the most common platform in use around the world today is the desktop or laptop PC.

A single platform shared among most of the world's businesses certainly has advantages – transmission and sharing of data between parties is easier and there is a large range of software suites that can be used. Also, support personnel do not need to specialize in certain types of system. There are also disadvantages, however, in that data become easier to steal, and 'malware' programs can affect a greater number of systems.

## The desktop PC – hardware

These machines are the 'backbone' of a veterinary practice network. They provide processing power for individual users, as well as access to resources and data. Connected to the PC are input devices, normally a keyboard and mouse, and an output device, which is normally a TFT LCD (thin film transistor liquid crystal display) monitor.

PCs have a modular construction; inside the case are separately identifiable components. The motherboard is the principal component of a PC system; this connects and synchronizes the other components, as well as providing sockets for connecting other devices. Into the motherboard is plugged the central processing unit (CPU). This is often thought of as the 'brain' of a computer, as it performs changes to the data passing through it, based on instructions that it receives from programs. Also plugged into the motherboard are memory modules, known as random-access memory (RAM) modules. This provides rapidly accessible short-term storage for programs and data (the RAM can only store data with power applied), and is where information and programs currently in use reside.

Another form of storage, which takes the physical appearance of a (normally silver) rectangular metal box, is the hard disk drive (HDD). This provides 'persistent' storage for programs and data, and has a greater storage capacity than the RAM. There is also a form of removable storage included in a PC base unit, normally a DVD-ROM drive, which allows data to be input and stored by the system for access by other PCs. The final component found inside a desktop PC is the power supply. This supplies the motherboard and other components with the power that they require to operate.

## The desktop PC – software

The most 'low level' software found on a PC is the basic input–output system, or BIOS. This provides the user with system set-up options, and provides the operating system (the next level of software) with a method to control the PC hardware.

The operating system (OS) is the most obvious piece of software to the user, as it provides an interface between the user and the hardware. The OS is responsible for managing the running of application programs, which may include office or accounting software, as well as the computer hardware. The application programs are often installed by end users, and are the programs that are required to make the computer truly useful. This is because they provide the specific functionality needed to complete a particular task or aspect of practice management. There is a vast range of PC applications available to complete almost every type of task.

## Networking

One major technology that has made computers even more useful is networking. This technology has been increasingly used by businesses with multiple computer systems since the 1980s, and today has become an essential aspect of computing in any business. Networks allow PCs and users to share resources. These may be data, programs, or items of hardware, such as storage devices and printers. Networks range from small networks of several computers in the home or office to the Internet, which is a worldwide network of PCs and smaller networks. Smaller networks are known as local area networks or LANs. A network spread over a larger geographical area is a wide area network, or WAN. A LAN is the type of network found in individual veterinary practice premises.

## Clients and servers

A server application is a program in control of a certain resource. Servers often provide a single source of data or item of hardware to many clients. In this respect, users in the practice running client programs on their desktop PCs are able to access the same resources without having to physically access the computer running the server application. A common use for the term 'server' is to describe the computer on which the server applications run. These large and expensive computers are required to provide service for up to thousands of users, and are not commonly found in individual practices. For a small-to-medium sized business, a standard desktop PC may be perfectly adequate as a server if there are a small number of workstations

(individual PCs) in use. Larger practices however, will often have larger, more specialized machines.

When a computer or device connects to a network, it is assigned a number called an IP address (IP stands for Internet Protocol). This number is unique to the device, and allows other users and devices to identify it on the network. It is through these numbers that network traffic arrives at the correct machine. The network traffic itself (another example of data) is sent in bursts known as 'packets'. Each packet of data contains the originating and destination IP addresses, the actual data to be transmitted, and error detecting and correcting information, so that the receiving machine can calculate whether the packet has been corrupted (altered) during transmission.

## Network Hardware

### Network interface controller (NIC)

More commonly known as a 'network card', this device is normally built into the PC as an integrated peripheral, although NICs can take other forms, such as USB 'dongles'. The purpose of the NIC is to provide a connection from a device to the network. Because of the widespread use of computer networks, most modern PCs and laptops now come with NICs built in to the motherboard.

## Cable

Network cable consists of four pairs of wire, with each pair twisted together. This configuration avoids interference with the network signals. The type of cable used is Category 5e, and this is terminated with small, rectangular plastic RJ45 plugs. Leads of this construction join the various networked devices to network switches. Category 5e cables can also terminate in wall sockets. In smaller practices, the other ends of the cables will plug into a network switch or router. The other ends of network cables in larger practices are often connected to a 'patch panel', which contains many (normally around 24) RJ45 sockets. These are then 'patched' via network cables to the required device, such as switch, router, or possibly a telephone line. Category 5e network cables can also be used to carry other forms of data, such as telephone signals. In larger installations, patch panels can be used to connect various parts of a network together in different locations.

## Switches

The network switch is the successor to the hub. Hubs were devices with multiple RJ45 sockets that connected all the sockets together. Because of this, all devices were able to 'listen' to all network traffic, and 'decide' which packets of data were intended for them. Switches are more advanced than hubs in that they dynamically make and break connections between RJ45 sockets. This allows only the data intended for a particular machine to reach it. A switch can be considered as a device for moving data between devices on a network. Switches can be quite small devices – with four to eight sockets, or larger rack mountable devices with up to 50 sockets.

## Routers

A router is a device that moves packets between computer networks. A router is the method by which a home or business network, such as the LAN in a practice, is connected to the Internet. The practice may also have a separate router for processing financial transactions. This is intended to increase security. Routers generally look quite similar, and are devices that resemble small network switches, but which also have a socket for a telephone line.

## Storage devices

These may take the form of a hard disk and power supply with a network connection, or of a dedicated file server PC. They are intended as central information stores for access by many clients on the network.

## Printers

Modern technology means that it is no longer necessary to have a dedicated PC as a print server, as many modern business printers have integrated NICs, and so can be directly plugged into the network. The set-up of network printers can often be conducted through an Internet browser application, or on the printer itself. Network printers can take many forms: from small A4 printers for normal office tasks, to photocopiers (which can often e-mail or fax scanned documents), to large-format printers for banner and poster printing.

## Telephones

Telephones can also be plugged into the network, as this allows for advanced features, such as call diverts for vets on call over weekends, the logging of calls, and advanced voicemail features, which are often hosted on a PC server. For this to operate with 'standard' or 'plain old telephone system' (POTS) telephones, small devices called public switched telephone network (PSTN) adaptors must be used on either end of a network cable, with a master phone socket on one end, and a telephone on the other. Using network infrastructure in this way is known as 'structured cabling'. Some systems assign IP addresses to each telephone on the network, and a further alternative is to use the network infrastructure to connect phones to a digital telephone exchange. This set-up is normally found in larger corporate practices and referral hospitals.

## Types of Malware

### Viruses

A virus can be written to disrupt service, to spread to as many machines as possible or merely to cause inconvenience, or a mixture of these. Many computer viruses have been reported on national news owing to the rate at which they spread, and the level of disruption that they cause. Viruses can be spread by many methods, but commonly they are spread as e-mail attachments or by being accidentally introduced into a network via an infected flash drive or CD-ROM. As the program code varies greatly between viruses, they can cause varying degrees of inconvenience. While one type of virus may simply cause a pop-up message to appear on affected PCs, others can cause damage to hardware and loss of data. Viruses, masquerading as legitimate files or programs, can also be downloaded by users.

### Trojans

A Trojan is named after the Trojan horse – it is a program that enters a system disguised as a legitimate application, and can be written for many purposes – to gather information, steal data, or aid in setting up a third-party attack, among others. Trojans can enter your system via similar methods to viruses – through e-mail attachments, downloaded from the Internet, or by individuals with physical access to the system.

## Root kits

Root kits consist of sets of small but powerful programs; which can be used by a third party to manipulate your computer in various ways. For example, such programs can be used to steal data or use your system to launch a third-party attack, such as a denial-of-service (DoS) attack. Users of root kits usually require a high level of access to your system before the root kit can be installed. Gaining access may be through an incorrectly configured firewall, or by having physical access to the system.

# Appendix 2
# Acceptable User Policy: Mobile and Landline Phones, E-mail and Internet

*<Practice Logo>*
<Practice Name>

## Staff Handbook

### Acceptable User Policy: Mobile and Landline Phones, E-mail and Internet

All staff are required to adhere to the following policy on the acceptable use of telephones, e-mail and the Internet when at work. The purpose of this policy is to protect you and the practice from any misuse of the practice's telecommunications systems. The practice may carry out monitoring of e-mail traffic, Internet and intranet use only for the purposes of ensuring security and the correct functioning of the network. Such monitoring will only be undertaken in accordance with a procedure agreed with all staff.

### Mobile phones

Use of mobile phones for personal calls should be restricted to breaks and lunchtimes only. However, it is recognized that from time to time there may be an emergency or you may need to take an urgent call. This limited use during working hours is permitted.

### Practice telephone system

Limited use of the practice telephones for personal reasons is permitted, excepting international calls.

### E-mail

Staff are expected to use e-mail for work-related purposes only. Please note that all e-mails sent to individuals and organizations outside the practice using the practice e-mail software carry the following disclaimer:

> This e-mail and any attachments are intended solely for the use of the individual to whom it is addressed. Any views or opinions expressed are solely those of the author and do not necessarily represent those of the <xxx> Veterinary Practice. If you are not the intended recipient, you must not act on its contents, copy it or show it to anyone. If you have received this e-mail in error, please contact the sender.

When using e-mail, all staff are required to adhere to the following rules:

- Keep your password secure and do not share it with anyone.
- Do not download or open attachments from an unknown source.
- Do not send confidential information via e-mail unless encrypted first, using the practice's encryption protocols.
- Always use appropriate e-mail etiquette when sending messages.
- Do not send or receive messages that may be harmful to any individual or any organization.
- Do not send messages that are illegal (e.g. discriminatory, sexist or racist, or which are in breach of copyright laws).
- Do not use the practice e-mail system for personal gain.

### Internet

Use of the Internet for work-related research is permitted and encouraged, but excessive use, which interferes with normal duties or with the functioning of the practice, is not permitted.

Anyone who wishes to use the Internet to distribute or share information or material of any kind in their capacity as a member of this practice must first seek permission from the Practice Manager to do so.

The practice web site, Facebook pages and Twitter are monitored and administered by the Practice Manager. Staff contributions are welcome and encouraged, but these must meet the practice's standards for acceptable content and quality.

Please note that an effective software firewall has been implemented across the network, which blocks access to unsafe or harmful web sites for your protection. If you have reason to believe that this protection is not functioning as it should, please contact the Practice Manager immediately.

## General conduct

Staff are expected to conduct themselves in a professional manner at all times and must not use the practice's telecommunications tools in a way that might harm the reputation of the practice, reveal confidential practice information to third parties, breach copyright laws, damage the practice network or otherwise harm the practice.

## Consequences of policy breaches

Any deliberate breaches of this policy will result in disciplinary action, which may lead to dismissal. The practice is obliged to report any illegal use of the practice computers and/or network to the appropriate authorities.

# Appendix 3
# Answers to Accounting Questions

## Chapter 17: The Profit and Loss Account

### Revision Question 1:

Sales = Sales – Sales returns
    = £165,000 – £25,000 = £140,000

Gross profit = Sales – Cost of sales
    = £140,000 – £15,000 = £125,000

Net profit = Gross profit – Expenses
    = £125,000 – £105,000 = £20,000

## Chapter 18: The Balance Sheet

### Question 1:

**Year 1:** June to September
(ignore part months) = 4 months

£15,000 × 0.17 = £2550 × 4/12
    = £850 depreciation
    for Year 1

£15,000 – £850 = £14,150 balance

**Year 2:**

£14,150 × 0.17 = £2406

£14,150 – £2406 = £11,744

**Year 3:**

£11,744 × 0.17 = £1996

£11,744 – £1996 = £9748

### Question 2:

Working capital = Total current assets – Total current liabilities

Total current assets = £15,000 (Stock)
    + £60,000 (Bank)
    + £500 (Cash)
    + £10,000 (Debtors)
    = £85,500

Total current liabilities = £600 (Creditors)
    + £1100 (Accrual)
    = £1700

Working capital = £85,500 – £1700
    = £83,800

### Question 4:

X and Y Current Accounts:

|  | X | Y |
|---|---|---|
| Opening balances at start of year | 35,000 | 45,000 |
| Salaries | 25,000 | 0 |
| Drawings | (6,000) | (10,000) |
|  | 54,000 | 35,000 |
| Share of net profit | 20,000 | 20,000 |
| Balances at year end | **74,000** | **55,000** |

## Chapter 19: Accounting Ratios and Financial Performance Indicators

### Question 2:

Average debtors = (£4500 + £6500) ÷ 2
    = £5500

Debtor days = (5500 ÷ 45,000) × 365 days
= 44.6 or 45 days,
approximately 1.5 months

## Chapter 20: Pricing, Products and Services

### Question 3:

Total annual costs = Overheads + Materials
+ Equipment
= £25,650 + £26,230 + £6,460
= £58,340 p.a.

£58,340 ÷ 1360 h = £42.90 p.h.

Cost of 1 h operation = Veterinarian time
+ Nurse time + Materials
+ Equipment
+ Overheads
= £35.65 + £15.00
+ £42.90 = £93.55

## Chapter 23: Evaluating Capital Investment

### Question 3:

| Year | 0 | 1 | 2 | 3 | 4 | 5 | 6 |
|---|---|---|---|---|---|---|---|
| Capital cost | (25,000) | | | | | | |
| Revenues | | 5,500 | 6,600 | 7,920 | 9,504 | 11,405 | 13,686 |
| Service contract | | (650) | (650) | (650) | (650) | (650) | (650) |
| **Net cash flow** | (25,000) | 4,850 | 5,950 | 7,270 | 8,854 | 10,755 | 13,036 |
| Discount factor | 1 | 0.91 | 0.83 | 0.75 | 0.68 | 0.62 | 0.56 |
| **Present value** | (25,000) | 4,414 | 4,939 | 5,453 | 6,021 | 6,668 | 7,300 |

Net present value = –£25,000 + £4414 + £4939 + £5453 + £6021 + £6668 + £7300 = £9795

# Index